ANSHI JAIN
NIMISH AGARWAL
NAKUL CHAUDHARY

FLUID AND ELECTROLYTE BALANCE IN POST- OPERATIVE SURGICAL PATIENTS

ANSHI JAIN
NIMISH AGARWAL
NAKUL CHAUDHARY

FLUID AND ELECTROLYTE BALANCE IN POST-OPERATIVE SURGICAL PATIENTS

LAP LAMBERT Academic Publishing

Cover image: www.ingimage.com

Publisher:
LAP LAMBERT Academic Publishing
is a trademark of
Dodo Books Indian Ocean Ltd. and OmniScriptum S.R.L publishing group

120 High Road, East Finchley, London, N2 9ED, United Kingdom
Str. Armeneasca 28/1, office 1, Chisinau MD-2012, Republic of Moldova, Europe
Managing Directors: Ieva Konstantinova, Victoria Ursu
info@omniscriptum.com

Printed at: see last page
ISBN: 978-620-8-43964-4

ACKNOWLEDGEMENT

It is with deep sense of gratitude, my thankful salutations to the Lord Almighty for giving me the time and inclination to complete this dissertation.

I would like to thank **Dr. Pradep Tangade** sir, Principal TMDC&RC for his constant support and for being a source of tremendous inspiration.

I extend my warmest thanks to **Dr. Nandakishore D.**, Professor and Head of the department of Oral and Maxillofacial Surgery Moradabad for his guidance and help in completing this Library dissertation with supreme sincerity and gratitude, I am deeply indebted for his complete support that I have been able to complete my dissertation in the stipulated time period.

I am extremely grateful to **Dr. D S Gupta**, Professor for their outsanding teaching, support and guidance and help all throughout.

I extend my warmest thanks to my guide **Dr. Nimish Agarwal**, Reader, of Oral and Maxillofacial Surgery for his guidance and help me in completing this Library dissertation With supreme sincerity and gratitude, It has been a privilege to prepare this dissertation under the able guidance of my revered teacher, who worked actively to provide me with the protected academic time to pursue my goals & had also helped me in compiling the enormous data of the study and without whom I could not have been able to finish my Library dissertation.

I extend my special thanks to **Dr. Akansh Datta, Dr. Saubhagya S. Agrawal, Dr. Sachin Dev** Reader, who has provided me extensive personal and professional guidance and taught me a great deal about both scientific research and life in general.

I am grateful to **Dr. Nakul Chaudhary** Senior Lecturer for providing me with the ideal academic environment for completing my dissertation.

Words would not be sufficient to express my deep sense of gratitude to my parents for their never ending, uninterrupted, unwavering and unconditional support. A special thanks to my parents **Mr. Pradeep Kumar Jain and Mrs. Deepali Jain** and my sister **Praptii Jain** for being a source of constant support and comfort to me at all times.

I also thank my seniors **Dr. Ali Qamar, Dr. Arghya Upadhyay, Dr. Mimansa Daftary, Dr. Shubham Mishra, Dr Upika Jain** batch mates **Dr. Raksha Sah, Dr. Subham, Dr. Kumari Aparajita and Dr. Anushka Singh** who had also helped me in compiling the enormous data of the study, and I thank them for their friendship, love, and unyielding support.

Each of the members of my Dissertation Committee has provided me extensive personal and professional guidance and taught me a great deal about both scientific research and life in general.

Lastly with deep sense of gratitude, I want to give thankful salutations to the Lord Almighty for giving me the time and inclination to complete this dissertation.

Dr. ANSHI JAIN

CONTENTS

LIST OF FIGURES

LIST OF ABBREVIATIONS

S. No.	Abbreviations	
1.	IV	Intravenous fluid
2.	ICF	Intracellular fluids
3.	ECF	Extracellular fluids
4.	ADH	Anti diuretic hormone
5.	ANP	Atrial natriuretic peptides
6.	DCT	Distal convoluted tubule
7.	CD	Collecting duct
8.	ACTH	Adreno Cortico Tropic Hormone
9.	RAAS	Renin-Angiotensin-Aldosterone-System

INTRODUCTION

Malnutrition has been used to describe a deficiency, excess or imbalance of a wide range of nutrients, resulting in a measurable adverse effect on body composition, function and clinical outcome. Malnutrition is a common, under-recognized and undertreated problem facing patients and clinicians. It is both a cause and consequence of disease and exists in institutional care and the community [1]. It occurs in about 30 per cent of surgical patients with gastrointestinal disease and in up to 60 per cent of those in whom hospital stay has been prolonged because of postoperative complications. It is frequently unrecognized and consequently patients often do not receive appropriate support [2]. Maintenance of normal fluid (water) balance is essential for the continuing functions of vital organs of body.

Electrolytes are essential for numerous bodily functions, including fluid balance, nerve and muscle function, pH regulation, and blood pressure control. Key electrolytes are sodium, potassium, calcium, magnesium, chloride, bicarbonate, and phosphate. Sodium (Na^+) controls fluid balance and blood pressure. It is also the key for nerve signals and muscle contractions. Potassium (K^+) is Crucial for maintaining normal cell function and fluid balance. It also plays a key role in muscle contractions and nerve signaling, particularly in the heart. Calcium (Ca^{2+}) is important for bone health and structure, and is necessary for muscle contraction, blood clotting, and nerve signaling. Magnesium (Mg^{2+}) is involved in over 300 biochemical reactions, including energy production. It supports muscle and nerve function, and helps regulate blood pressure. Chloride (Cl^-) helps maintain fluid balance and osmotic pressure. It is important for the production of stomach acid (HCl), which aids digestion.

Typically, the concentration of electrolytes inside cells differs from that in plasma. The body maintains normal serum electrolyte levels through a careful balance of four processes: intake, absorption, distribution, and excretion. Disruptions in any of these processes due to various health conditions can lead to electrolyte imbalances. Precise perioperative management of fluids and electrolytes is a fundamental part of a patient's overall surgical treatment, which can have a significant effect on perioperative morbidity and mortality [3]. Ensuring sufficient preoperative stabilization before administering general anesthesia is essential to prevent complications such as hypotension, renal failure, cardiac dysrhythmias, and other potential issues during surgery.

Intravenous fluid (IV) therapy is a cornerstone to treating shock status and providing water, electrolytes and glucose needs. The appropriate use of IV fluids is an essential part of patient safety and deserves careful oversight and guidance, given the association between fluid (mis)use and the deleterious effects causing patient morbidity and mortality [4]. Proper fluid and electrolyte management during the postoperative and convalescent periods will depend to a great extent upon the patient's preoperative status and preparation, the magnitude of surgical trauma, and the fluids administered intraoperatively [5]. In the past, patients undergoing major surgery were often administered large volumes of crystalloid, based on a presumption of preoperative dehydration and nebulous intraoperative 'third space' fluid loss. However, positive perioperative fluid balance, with postoperative fluid-based weight gain, is associated with increased major morbidity. A 'restrictive' fluid approach during surgery—where fluid is limited to just what is needed to avoid low blood volume—initially showed a reduction in major complications after complex surgeries. However, variations in what is considered 'restrictive' versus 'liberal' fluid use, the types of fluids given, and how complications are defined have led to mixed results in clinical trials. Managing fluid resuscitation for patients after surgery remains a continual challenge, with ongoing reviews and debates leading to evolving recommendations about which fluids to use—whether crystalloids, colloids, packed red blood cells, fresh whole blood, or clotting factors [1]. Additionally, factors like the availability of resources can influence the choice of fluids made by healthcare practitioners. Achieving balance in the resuscitation period is challenging, particularly the volume administered. Administration of more fluid is not always correct. Much of the literature on fluid resuscitation focuses on critically ill patients with sepsis, or elective perioperative patients. To improve care of comprehensive patient, oral and maxillofacial surgeons require a sound knowledge of the basic principles of fluid management and use a sound strategy for blood product usage [6].

The fundamental goal of perioperative fluid management is on one hand—to achieve a balance between avoiding hypotension, impaired tissue oxygenation, and inadequate organ profusion that may be associated with too little fluid, and—on the other hand—to avoid interstitial edema and cardiopulmonary complications associated with fluid overload [7]

The discussion starts with determining the number of fluids to be given before, during, and after surgery. Historically, this decision has relied on the surgeon's clinical judgment. Maintenance fluid requirements are roughly estimated based on insensible and obligatory losses. Several formulas exist to calculate fluid replacement, often using a patient's weight or surface area.

NICE guidelines recommend 25-30 ml/kg/day of fluid and 1 mmol/kg/day of sodium, potassium, and chloride [8].

The rationale of this dissertation is to review the literature about the fluid and electrolyte balance in surgical patients.

HISTORICAL BACKGROUND

The history of fluid and electrolyte balance can be traced through various key developments in medicine and science:

1. **Ancient Understanding**:
   - Ancient civilizations recognized the importance of water for health. Hippocrates (c. 460–370 BC) emphasized the role of fluids in bodily functions, although the specific understanding of electrolytes was limited.
2. **17th Century**:
   - In the 1600s, William Harvey's work on blood circulation highlighted the importance of maintaining fluid balance in the body.
3. **19th Century**:
   - The development of chemistry and physiology began to shed light on the role of minerals in the body. Scientists identified sodium, potassium, and chloride as key electrolytes.
4. **20th Century**:
   - The concept of homeostasis, introduced by Walter Cannon in the early 1900s, explained how the body maintains internal stability, including fluid and electrolyte balance.
   - Rudolph Matas in 1924 first proposed the administration of an intravenous 'drip' during surgery and this has been validated and advanced manifold since then by Moore and Shires in the 1940s and 1950s and by Shoemaker in the 1970s.
   - The Holliday-Segar method was introduced in 1957 by Dr Holliday and Dr Segar to provide a systematic way to calculate fluid requirements in children.
   - The discovery of hormones like aldosterone and antidiuretic hormone (ADH) in the mid-20th century clarified their roles in regulating fluid and electrolyte balance.

5. **Modern Medicine**:
    - Advances in medical technology allowed for better measurement of electrolyte levels in blood and urine, leading to improved diagnosis and treatment of imbalances.
    - Research into conditions like dehydration, heart failure, and kidney disease deepened understanding of how electrolyte balance affects health.

Overall, the study of fluid and electrolyte balance has evolved from basic observations about water and health to a complex understanding of biochemical processes and their implications for medical science.

REVIEW OF LITERATURE

1. **Tom Shires et al (1961)** [9] explores the impact of major surgeries on extracellular fluid dynamics. It reviews how surgical interventions can cause significant shifts in extracellular fluid compartments, affecting patient hemodynamics and recovery. The article emphasizes the need for careful monitoring and management of fluid balance to mitigate complications such as hypovolemia or edema. By analyzing various studies and clinical data, the authors highlight the importance of understanding fluid shifts to improve surgical outcomes and patient safety.

2. **Robert W. Virtue et al (1965)** [10] investigated how different intravenous fluids—glucose, saline, and lactate—affect fluid distribution and shifts during surgery. By utilizing RISA (radioactive iodinated serum albumin) and sodium determinations, the research provides insights into the dynamics of fluid compartments and their responses to various infusion solutions. The findings offer valuable guidance on selecting appropriate fluids to manage intraoperative fluid balance effectively and optimize patient outcomes.

3. **A.I. Mackenzie et al (1969)** [11] examine the intricate relationship between urine output and fluid management in the perioperative setting. The article explores how urine output serves as a critical indicator of fluid status and renal function during surgery and anesthesia. The authors review various strategies for fluid therapy, including the administration of crystalloids and colloids, and their impact on urine output and overall patient stability. They emphasize the importance of monitoring urine output to guide fluid management decisions and adjust treatment in real-time. The paper synthesizes findings from both historical and recent studies, highlighting the evolution of fluid management practices and their implications for minimizing complications. Mackenzie and Donald advocate for a balanced approach to fluid therapy that considers both the volume of fluids administered and the physiological responses of the patient. Their review provides valuable

insights for optimizing perioperative fluid management to enhance patient outcomes and reduce the risk of renal and circulatory complications.

4. **Jenkins et al (1975)** [12] offer a comprehensive analysis of fluid and electrolyte management in postoperative care. They emphasize the critical role of tailored fluid resuscitation strategies to maintain hemodynamic stability and support recovery, detailing the use of crystalloids versus colloids based on patient-specific factors. The article highlights common postoperative electrolyte imbalances such as hyponatremia and hyperkalemia, advocating for vigilant monitoring and prompt correction. Jenkins et al. stress the importance of individualized care plans, reflecting advances in understanding postoperative physiology and management. Their findings build on earlier research by Holliday and Segar, integrating modern approaches and technologies for enhanced patient outcomes. This article is a valuable resource for clinicians seeking to optimize fluid and electrolyte management in diverse postoperative scenarios, underscoring the need for personalized treatment strategies.

5. **Birgitte Brandstrup et al (2003)** [13] evaluated the impact of fluid restriction versus more liberal fluid regimens on postoperative outcomes. The study provides evidence that restrictive fluid therapy can reduce postoperative complications, such as wound infections and respiratory issues, compared to liberal fluid administration. It highlights the benefits of a controlled fluid regimen in improving recovery and reducing adverse effects. The research underscores the importance of tailored fluid management strategies in enhancing patient outcomes and minimizing complications in the postoperative period.

6. **Finfer et al (2004)** [14] evaluates the efficacy of albumin versus saline for fluid resuscitation in the intensive care unit, based on the SAFE Study. Published in 2004 in the *New England Journal of Medicine*, this study compares the outcomes of patients receiving either albumin or saline, revealing no significant difference in mortality or major complications between the two fluids. The review highlights that while both fluids are effective, the choice of resuscitation fluid

should be guided by individual patient needs and specific clinical circumstances. The study underscores the ongoing debate in critical care regarding the optimal fluid for resuscitation and emphasizes the need for continued research to refine fluid management practices.

7. **SAFE Study Investigators (2004)** [15] critically evaluated the efficacy of albumin versus saline for fluid resuscitation in critically ill patients. The research highlights that while albumin may offer some advantages in specific clinical scenarios, overall outcomes between albumin and saline are similar, suggesting that saline remains a cost-effective option for fluid resuscitation. This study provides valuable insights into optimizing fluid management strategies in intensive care settings, emphasizing the need for individualized patient care.

8. **C. H. Maharaj et al (2005)** [16] examined the effects of preoperative intravenous fluid administration on postoperative outcomes. Their research demonstrates that such therapy significantly reduces postoperative nausea and pain, particularly in high-risk patients. The study supports the use of preoperative fluid optimization as a strategy to enhance recovery and improve patient comfort following surgery.

9. **Barbara Kabon et al (2005)** [17] examines the effectiveness of additional crystalloid fluid administration in preventing surgical wound infections. The findings indicate that increased intravenous crystalloid volumes do not significantly impact the incidence of wound infections in surgical patients. This literature underscores the need for reevaluating fluid management strategies in the context of infection prevention, suggesting that factors other than fluid volume may be more critical in reducing postoperative infection risk.

10. **Lobo et al (2006)** [18] Provides a thorough examination of the impact of fluid balance on recovery and postoperative complications. The article reviews how both fluid overload and deficit can adversely affect surgical outcomes, emphasizing the role of precise perioperative fluid management in minimizing complications. The authors analyze recent studies and clinical trials to highlight

the benefits of goal-directed fluid therapy and individualized fluid management strategies. They discuss the relationship between fluid balance and key postoperative factors, such as wound healing, infection rates, and organ function. The review integrates current best practices and evidence-based guidelines, advocating for real-time monitoring and adjustment of fluid therapy to optimize patient recovery. By synthesizing past research and recent advancements, the article offers valuable insights into improving perioperative care and enhancing patient outcomes through effective fluid management.

11. **Daniel Chappell et al (2008)** [19] Offers a comprehensive review of fluid management strategies in the perioperative setting. It emphasizes a balanced approach, integrating both evidence-based practices and physiological principles to guide fluid therapy. The authors critique various fluid types and administration protocols, advocating for a personalized strategy based on patient-specific factors and surgical demands. They also discuss the importance of monitoring and adjusting fluid therapy to prevent complications and enhance recovery, reflecting a nuanced understanding of fluid dynamics in major surgeries.

12. **Price et al (2008)** [20] provides a comprehensive analysis of perioperative fluid volume management in patients with proximal femoral fractures. The authors highlight the critical role of fluid optimization in enhancing surgical outcomes and reducing complications. They discuss various fluid management strategies, emphasizing the need for individualized approaches based on patient-specific factors and surgical contexts. This review underscores the importance of balancing fluid administration to achieve optimal hemodynamic stability and recovery.

13. **Zubin M. Bamboat et al (2009)** [21] provides an in-depth review of strategies for fluid management throughout the perioperative period. It examines various fluid types, including crystalloids and colloids, and their roles in optimizing patient outcomes during and after surgery. The review discusses the balance between avoiding fluid overload and ensuring adequate hydration, as well as the impact of

goal-directed fluid therapy (GDFT) on recovery and complication rates. The authors also highlight the importance of personalized fluid management approaches tailored to individual patient needs and surgical contexts.

14. **Mike S. Strunden et al (2011)** [22] provides a thorough review of the principles and practices of fluid management during the perioperative period. The paper explores the physiological foundations underlying fluid balance and evaluates various tools and strategies used to optimize volume management. By integrating recent advancements and evidence-based approaches, the study offers a comprehensive framework for enhancing patient care and improving surgical outcomes through effective fluid management.

15. **Doherty et al (2012)** [23] review on intraoperative fluid management examines the risks and benefits associated with fluid administration during surgery. They highlight the challenges in determining optimal fluid volumes, noting that excessive fluid can lead to complications like edema and impaired recovery, while inadequate fluid may result in inadequate perfusion. The review emphasizes the need for personalized fluid management strategies and careful monitoring to balance these risks effectively.

16. **Sean M. Bagshaw et al (2012)** [24] critically evaluate the use of hydroxyethyl starch (HES) in managing fluid resuscitation among critically ill patients. Their review highlights the efficacy of HES in improving hemodynamic stability but also discusses associated risks and complications, such as renal impairment. The study underscores the need for cautious use and individualized patient assessment to balance benefits and potential harms in critical care settings.

17. **John A. Myburgh et al (2013)** [25] provides a comprehensive overview of contemporary practices and advances in critical care. Finfer and Vincent's work offers a broad perspective on critical care principles and management strategies, while Myburgh and Mythen delve into the specifics of resuscitation fluid therapy, addressing the latest research on fluid types and administration techniques.

Together, these texts underscore the dynamic nature of critical care medicine and the ongoing evolution of evidence-based practices.

18. **Jeffrey L. Carson et al (2013)** [26] investigates the impact of transfusion strategies on outcomes in patients with coronary artery disease. The research demonstrates that a restrictive transfusion threshold, compared to a liberal approach, is associated with similar or even better clinical outcomes, including reduced mortality and fewer complications. This literature emphasizes the potential benefits of adopting a more conservative transfusion strategy, challenging traditional practices and highlighting the need for tailored transfusion protocols in managing symptomatic coronary artery disease.

19. **Càndid Villanueva et al (2013)** [27] explores the impact of different blood transfusion approaches on outcomes in patients with acute upper gastrointestinal bleeding. It highlights evidence that more conservative transfusion strategies, such as targeting higher hemoglobin thresholds, can be as effective as liberal transfusion practices and may reduce complications and resource use. This literature underscores the importance of personalized transfusion protocols to enhance patient outcomes and optimize clinical management in acute bleeding scenarios.

20. **Caironi et al (2014)** [28] highlights the complex role of albumin as a fluid resuscitation strategy. The study provides insights into the effectiveness of albumin compared to crystalloids, with evidence suggesting potential benefits in terms of reducing mortality and improving hemodynamic stability. However, the review also underscores the need for further research to optimize treatment protocols and fully understand the implications of albumin use in critical care settings.

21. **Hong Jin Shim (2014)** [29] the effect of maintaining a positive fluid balance on outcomes in critically ill noncardiac postsurgical patients is explored through a retrospective cohort design. The literature suggests that positive fluid balance can

lead to various complications, including increased mortality and longer hospital stays. However, Shim's findings indicate a potential association between positive fluid balance and improved clinical outcomes in certain patient subsets, challenging conventional views. This study adds to the ongoing discourse on fluid management strategies in critical care, emphasizing the need for individualized approaches. Future research should focus on prospective trials to better delineate the impact of fluid balance on recovery trajectories in this vulnerable population.

22. **Ettinger et al.'s (2014)** [30] study investigates how intraoperative fluid administration affects the length of postoperative hospital stay following orthognathic surgery. The literature review reveals that both the volume and type of fluids administered can significantly influence recovery times. The authors found that more precise fluid management correlates with shorter hospital stays, highlighting the importance of optimizing fluid strategies to improve postoperative outcomes in orthognathic procedures.

23. **Kayilioglu, Dinc et al (2015)** [31] provides a comprehensive overview of current strategies and considerations in managing fluids after surgery. The article discusses the critical balance required in postoperative fluid management to prevent both overload and dehydration, emphasizing the role of individualized fluid therapy based on patient-specific factors and surgical complexity. The authors review various fluid types, including crystalloids and colloids, and their impact on recovery and complication rates. They highlight the importance of monitoring techniques and decision-making tools that guide fluid administration and adjustment throughout the postoperative period. The paper also explores the latest evidence on goal-directed fluid therapy and its benefits in enhancing recovery and reducing adverse outcomes. By integrating findings from recent research and clinical practice, Kayilioglu et al. offer practical insights and recommendations for optimizing fluid management to improve postoperative results and patient safety.

24. **Saraghi's (2015)** [32] review on intraoperative fluids and fluid management in ambulatory dental sedation and general anesthesia addresses the nuanced requirements of fluid administration in these settings. The literature underscores the importance of careful fluid balance to minimize complications and optimize patient outcomes. Saraghi highlights that while adequate hydration is crucial, excessive fluid can lead to adverse effects, emphasizing the need for tailored fluid management strategies based on individual patient needs and procedural demands.

25. **F. Hariri et al (2016)** [33] analyze the principles of fluid management specific to oral and maxillofacial surgical procedures. Their review emphasizes the importance of tailored fluid strategies to address the unique challenges and physiological responses in these surgeries. By reassessing fluid management protocols, the study aims to optimize patient outcomes and minimize complications in oral and maxillofacial surgical contexts.

26. **Robert Wise et al (2017)** [34] explores optimal fluid resuscitation techniques for trauma patients, focusing on the balance between efficacy and safety. The review examines various intravenous fluid strategies and their impact on outcomes such as hemodynamic stability and organ function. Emphasizing evidence-based practices, the study underscores the importance of tailored resuscitation approaches to improve survival and recovery in trauma settings.

27. **Christina H. Shin et al (2017)** [35] analyze the impact of intraoperative fluid management strategies on postoperative recovery. Their study, utilizing hospital registry data, highlights how different fluid management practices can significantly influence postoperative outcomes such as recovery time and complication rates. The findings underscore the critical role of optimizing fluid management during surgery to improve patient outcomes and inform best practices in clinical settings

28. **Makaryus et al (2018)** [36] provides a detailed review of contemporary fluid management strategies within enhanced recovery protocols. The article highlights

the shift from traditional, aggressive fluid resuscitation methods to more balanced approaches that emphasize optimal fluid balance to reduce postoperative complications. The authors discuss how individualized fluid management, guided by patient-specific factors and real-time monitoring, enhances recovery and minimizes adverse outcomes. They review current evidence supporting goal-directed fluid therapy and the use of advanced monitoring technologies to refine fluid administration. The paper integrates findings from recent clinical trials and studies, showing how these approaches align with the broader goals of enhanced recovery pathways. Makaryus et al. also address the importance of multimodal analgesia and early mobilization in conjunction with fluid management strategies. Their review underscores the evolving landscape of postoperative care and provides practical insights for improving patient outcomes through refined fluid management practices.

29. **Dongho Kang et al (2019)** [37] reviews contemporary approaches to fluid management in both surgical and critical care settings. The paper highlights key strategies for optimizing fluid therapy to enhance patient outcomes, focusing on the balance between avoiding fluid overload and ensuring adequate tissue perfusion. Their comprehensive review emphasizes the importance of individualized fluid management protocols and the need for ongoing research to refine these practices in varied clinical scenarios.

30. **Timothy E. Miller et al (2019)** [38] offers a thorough review of fluid management strategies for major surgical procedures. It examines various types of fluids, including crystalloids and colloids, and discusses the principles behind goal-directed fluid therapy (GDFT). The review highlights the benefits and limitations of different fluid strategies, such as liberal versus restrictive approaches, and emphasizes evidence supporting individualized fluid management to improve patient outcomes. Recent advances and ongoing controversies in the field are also addressed, with a focus on refining practices and integrating new monitoring technologies.

31. **N. Heming et al (2019)** [39] explore perioperative fluid management strategies for major elective surgery, emphasizing the critical balance between maintaining adequate hydration and preventing complications such as fluid overload. They analyze various fluid administration protocols, including goal-directed therapy and the use of balanced crystalloids versus colloids, highlighting the importance of individualized approaches based on patient-specific factors. The authors underscore the role of enhanced recovery after surgery (ERAS) protocols in optimizing fluid management and improving postoperative outcomes. Additionally, they call for further research to establish standardized guidelines that can enhance safety and efficacy in fluid administration during the perioperative period.

32. **Birgitte Brandstrup et al (2019)** [40] reviewed literature on the challenge of perioperative fluid management in elderly patients highlights the complexities of hydration strategies in this vulnerable population. It emphasizes that age-related physiological changes, comorbidities, and altered kidney function necessitate careful fluid administration to avoid complications such as fluid overload or dehydration. The review advocates for personalized approaches, integrating monitoring technologies and evidence-based guidelines to optimize outcomes while minimizing risks. Brandstrup calls for further research to refine fluid management protocols tailored to the unique needs of elderly patients.

33. **Christian J. Wiedermann (2020)** [41] explores the evolving strategies of fluid management, emphasizing the integral role of human albumin solution. Wiedermann reviews its efficacy in stabilizing hemodynamics and improving outcomes during critical and perioperative care, highlighting both the benefits and limitations of albumin use. The literature underscores the importance of tailored fluid management approaches and the potential impact of albumin in optimizing patient recovery and survival.

34. **Manu L. N. G. Malbrain et al (2020)** [42] provide a comprehensive overview of best practices for fluid management in perioperative and critical care

environments. The summary synthesizes current guidelines and evidence on fluid therapy, addressing key strategies to optimize patient outcomes and minimize complications. This executive summary reflects a consensus on the importance of individualized fluid management approaches and the need for ongoing research to refine these practices.

35. **R.K. Kamel et al (2021)** [43] reviews emerging strategies and innovations in managing fluids during the perioperative period. It discusses advancements in fluid types, including the use of balanced crystalloids and the role of goal-directed fluid therapy in improving surgical outcomes. The review highlights the shift towards personalized fluid management approaches that consider individual patient factors and surgical variables to optimize fluid balance and minimize complications. It also emphasizes the importance of integrating new monitoring technologies and evidence-based practices to enhance perioperative care.

36. **Atte Koskinen et al (2023)** [44] investigate the incidence and implications of postoperative fluid accumulation in cardiac surgery patients. The study identifies key factors contributing to fluid retention and its impact on recovery and outcomes. The authors emphasize the need for vigilant fluid management strategies to mitigate risks and enhance postoperative care. Their findings contribute valuable insights into optimizing fluid therapy to prevent complications and improve patient outcomes following cardiac surgery.

37. **Hahn et al (2023)** [45] explore the intricate dynamics between nonfinancial reporting and genuine sustainability transformations in organizations. The authors critique current reporting practices, suggesting that while they aim to promote transparency, they often fall short of driving meaningful change. They emphasize the need for a deeper understanding of how these reports influence stakeholder behavior and corporate strategies. Through their analysis, the authors highlight the complexities involved in aligning reporting with actual sustainable practices, advocating for a more integrated approach that goes beyond mere compliance.

This work contributes to the ongoing dialogue on sustainability in business, questioning the effectiveness of reporting as a tool for real impact.

38. **Sharnice Koek et al. (2024)** [46] reviews fluid management strategies specifically for patients undergoing pancreaticoduodenectomy within the enhanced recovery after surgery (ERAS) framework. It evaluates various postoperative fluid protocols and their impact on recovery outcomes, such as complications, length of hospital stays, and overall patient well-being. The review highlights the benefits of tailored fluid therapy in reducing postoperative complications and supporting quicker recovery, while addressing ongoing debates about optimal fluid volume and type. The authors emphasize the need for individualized approaches and evidence-based guidelines to improve patient outcomes in this high-risk surgical population.

39. **Hahn et al (2024)** [47] critically assess the National Institute for Health and Care Excellence (NICE) guidelines, highlighting the potential limitations and inconsistencies in the recommendations for maintenance fluid therapy. They argue that while the guidelines aim to standardize care, there are gaps in evidence that could affect patient outcomes. The authors call for a more nuanced approach that considers individual patient needs and underlying conditions. Their analysis underscores the importance of ongoing research to refine fluid therapy protocols and improve clinical practice. This review contributes to the broader discourse on optimizing patient care in hospital settings, emphasizing the need for guidelines to be both evidence-based and adaptable.

40. **Hahn et al (2023)** [48] explore the intricate dynamics between nonfinancial reporting and genuine sustainability transformations in organizations. The authors critique current reporting practices, suggesting that while they aim to promote transparency, they often fall short of driving meaningful change. They emphasize the need for a deeper understanding of how these reports influence stakeholder behavior and corporate strategies. Through their analysis, the authors highlight the complexities involved in aligning reporting with actual sustainable practices,

advocating for a more integrated approach that goes beyond mere compliance. This work contributes to the ongoing dialogue on sustainability in business, questioning the effectiveness of reporting as a tool for real impact.

41. **Indunil Karunarathna et al. (2024)** [49] offers a comprehensive overview of fluid management approaches essential for critically ill patients. The authors emphasize the importance of individualized fluid therapy, considering factors such as patient condition, underlying diseases, and response to treatment. They review various strategies, including the use of dynamic parameters for fluid responsiveness and the role of balanced crystalloids versus saline. The paper also highlights the risks of fluid overload and the need for careful monitoring to prevent complications. Overall, the article serves as a valuable resource for clinicians aiming to enhance patient outcomes through effective fluid management in critical care settings.

DISCUSSION

An appreciation of the distribution of water (the aqueous biological solvent) and its solutes is fundamental to understanding the physiology of body fluid spaces. Traditionally blood has been treated as an intravascular fluid circulation, while the lymphatic vessels have been called a drainage system. The modern view is of an actively pumped double circulation of extracellular fluid (intravascular plasma, and interstitial fluid and lymph) that enables vital solutes to be transferred to and from the intracellular fluid. Fluid flux across cell membrane barriers and across the different microvascular permeability barriers is determined by hydrostatic pressure differences and solute concentration gradients. Total body water volume is largely regulated by the pituitary hormonal effect of arginine vasopressin acting on vasopressin type 2 receptors in renal collecting ducts to retain or release water. In critical illness, arginine vasopressin deficiency predisposes patients to dilutional hyponatremia if the infused volume is larger than necessary or excessively prescribed as 'electrolyte-free water'. Evidence from surgical practice suggests that adaptive mechanisms exist to stabilize the intracellular volume in the face of excessive intravenous fluid infusions, and an alternative model of body water response to intravenous infusions is proposed [3].

TOTAL BODY WATER

The body water accounts for 60% of body weight in young adult male & 50% for young females. A normal variation of (+/-5) % is applied to both groups. The total body water is highest in the new born infants, which constitutes 77% of body weight. The water content falls rapidly during first 6 months of life to below 65% & more slowly during the next years on an average to 59%. Fat contains little water, so thin individual has a greater portion of water to body weight than the obese individual. The lower percentage of total body water in females correlates with the relatively large amount of subcutaneous fat & less muscle mass. An extremely obese individual may have 25 to 35% less body water than a thin individual of same weight [50]. The correct degree of retention & expulsion to establish a normal balance is accompanied by kidney function.

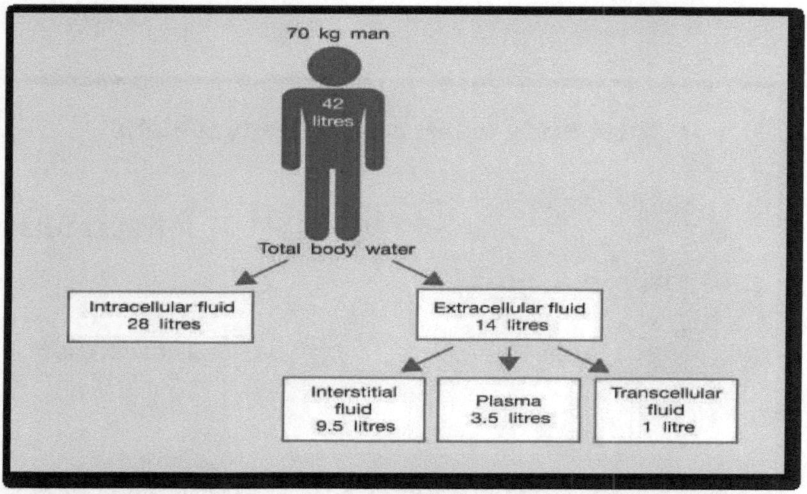

Figure 1 – Compartmentalisation of total body water in an average 70kg man

Courtesy- Henderson MA, Gillon S, Al-Haddad M. Organization and composition of body fluids. Anaesthesia & Intensive Care Medicine. 2021 Aug 1;22(8):511-7

BODY FLUIDS

Body fluids are made up of water, salts, blood plasma, cells, proteins, and other substances that dissolve in liquids. They are located in two main areas inside the body: inside the cells (intracellular) and outside the cells (extracellular) [1].

Intracellular fluids (ICF) are found inside cells and are made up of protein, water, electrolytes, and solutes. The most abundant electrolyte in intracellular fluid is potassium. Intracellular fluid accounts for 60% of the volume of body fluids and 40% of a person's total body weight [10]. This water forms part of protoplasm of the cells & is distributed in many small compartments or cell separated from each other by two cell membranes & layer of interstitial fluid. Potassium & magnesium, are the principal cations, whereas the phosphates & proteins are the principal anions in intracellular fluids. The largest portion of this is intracellular water is with in skeletal muscle mass [1].

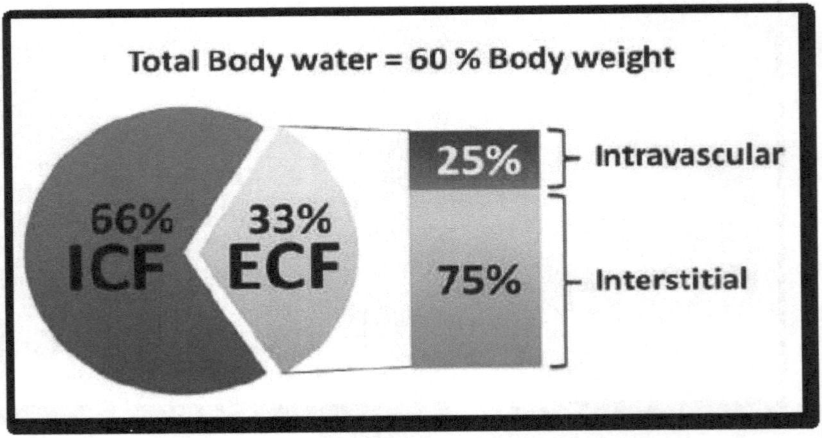

Figure 2 - Total body water

Courtesy- Stanzani G, Chan DL. Controversies in fluid therapy. European Journal of Companion Animal Practice. 2010;24(2).

Extracellular fluids (ECF) are fluids found outside of cells. The most abundant electrolyte in extracellular fluid is sodium. The body regulates sodium levels to control the movement of water into and out of the extracellular space due to osmosis [51].

Extracellular fluids are further broken down into various types-

a) Intravascular fluid – It is situated within blood vessels constitute 7%. It is whole blood volume and also includes red blood cells, white blood cells, plasma, and platelets. Intravascular fluid is the most important part of the body's fluid balance.
b) Interstitial or extracellular fluid – It is the fluid that lies outside of blood vessels and between the cells. It constitutes 17% of total body water. The most abundant electrolyte in extracellular fluid is sodium. The body regulates

sodium levels to control the movement of water into and out of the extracellular space due to osmosis. Excess of interstitial fluids is known as edema.

c) Transcellular fluid – It includes fluid which is extravascular but not interstitial. It is the fluid in areas like cerebrospinal, synovial, intrapleural and gastrointestinal system.[2]

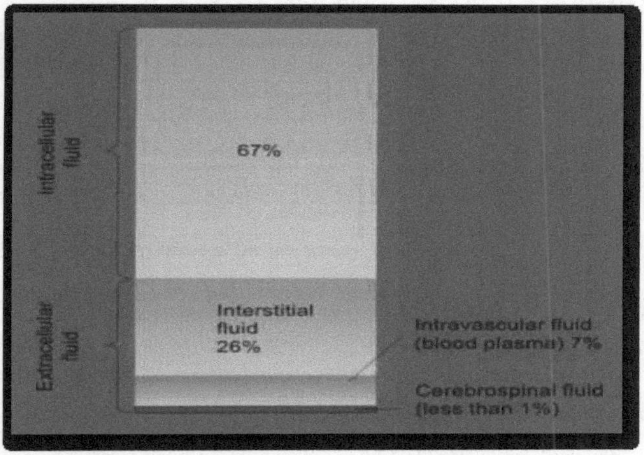

Figure 3 - Intracellular and Extracellular Components

Courtesy- Open Resources for Nursing (Open RN); Ernst Meyer K, Christman E, editors. Nursing Fundamentals [Internet]. Eau Claire (WI): Chippewa Valley Technical College; 2021. Chapter 15 Fluids and Electrolytes.

Marker Substances:

Used to measure volumes of body fluid compartments.

COMPARTMENT	MARKER SUBSTANCE
TOTAL BODY WATER	D_2O (Deuterium oxide), H_3O (Titrated water), Antipyrine
EXTRACELLULAR	Radioisotopes of selected ions (Na+, Cl^-, Br^-, SO_4, S_2O_3), Nonmetabolizable saccharides like insulin, mannitol, raffinose
PLASMA	Evans blue dye
INTRACELLULAR FLUID	It is measured by subtracting the extracellular fluid from measured total body water.

Fluid intake is derived from both exogenous (consumed liquids) and endogenous (released during oxidation of solid foodstuffs) fluids.[2]

The average daily water balance of a healthy adult is shown in Table-

OUTPUT	VOLUME (ml)	INTAKE	VOLUME (ml)
Urine	1500	Water from beverage	200
Insensible losses	900	Water from food	1000
Faeces	100	Water from oxidation	300

Courtesy- Bailey H, Love R. Chapter 20: Nutrition and fluid therapy. In: Bailey H, Love R, editors. Bailey and Love's Short Practice of Surgery. 26th ed. London: Hodder Arnold; 2013. p. [261-271]

Fluid losses occur by four routes –

1) Lungs- Approximately 400 mL of water is lost through expired air every 24 hours. This loss is greater in dry environments or for patients with a tracheostomy, highlighting the need to humidify the inhaled air.
2) Skin- In a temperate climate, skin (i.e. sweat) losses are between 600 and 1000 mL/day.
3) Faeces - Between 60 and 150 mL of water are lost daily in patients with normal bowel function.
4) Urine - The typical urine output is around 1500 mL per day, and when the kidneys are functioning properly, the specific gravity of urine is directly related to its volume. To effectively eliminate the byproducts of protein metabolism, a minimum urine output of 400 mL per day is necessary.[2]

NORMAL EXCHANGE OF FLUID AND ELECTROLYTES

I) WATER

Intake-

a) Exogenous Sources

Water from beverage – 1200ml

Water from solid food - 1000ml

b) Endogenous Sources

Water from oxidation – 300ml

Output-

Urine mainly controlled by ADH - 1500 ml

Insensible loss from skin & lungs -900 ml

Faeces-100 ml

It must be remembered that water requirements of children are relatively larger than those of adults as

o Water content is higher in respect to total body weight.

o Metabolic activity is greater in children due to growth.

o Immature kidneys of children are poor in concentrating ability.

The following are the approximate daily requirements of some electrolytes in adults [1]:

• sodium: 50–90 mM/day;

• potassium: 50 mM/day;

• calcium: 5 mM/day;

• magnesium: 1 mM/day

The nature and type of fluid replacement therapy will be determined by individual patient needs.

Table 3 [1]- Composition of crystalloid and colloid solutions(mmol/L)-

SOLUTION	Na	K	Ca	Cl	LACTATE	COLLOID
Hartmann's	131	5	21	111	29	
Normal Saline (0.9% NaCl)	154	154				
Dextrose saline (4% dextrose in 0.19% saline)	30	30				
Gelofusine	150	150				Gelatin 4%
Haemacel	145	5.1	<1	145		Polygelin 75g/L Hydroxyethyl starch 6%
Hetastarch						

In addition to maintenance requirements, 'replacement' fluids are required to correct pre-existing deficiencies and 'supplemental' fluids are required to compensate for anticipated additional intestinal or other losses [1]. The nature and volumes of these fluids are determined by-

i) A thorough evaluation of the patient should include checking the pulse, blood pressure, and, if possible, central venous pressure. The clinical examination should focus on assessing hydration levels through examination of extremities, skin turgor, urine output, and the specific gravity of urine. Additionally, urine and serum electrolytes, as well as hematocrit levels, should be measured.

ii) Assessing the types and extent of losses that have occurred, such as those from vomiting, ileus, diarrhea, excessive sweating, or fluid loss due to burns or severe inflammatory conditions.

iii) Estimating the additional fluids that will likely be needed based on expected future losses from drains, fistulas, nasogastric tubes, or abnormal urine and fecal output.

iv) Once the required fluid volumes have been estimated, the suitable replacement fluid can be chosen by evaluating the electrolyte content of gastrointestinal secretions. Typically, most intestinal losses can be effectively replaced with normal saline supplemented with potassium. [3]

ROLE OF WATER

Control of Extracellular Fluid Osmolality & Sodium Concentration

The various mechanisms are:

1. **Arterial baroreceptor & atrial natriuretic factor**

This acts on kidneys actively to increase Na & water excretion to as much as 3- 10-fold. Atrial natriuretic peptides (ANP) are released from the atria upon stretching and play a major role in the control of sodium and fluid balance. The decrease in alpha-ANP was associated with a decline in cardiac index, creatinine clearance, urinary output and urinary sodium excretion. The reasons behind the decline in release of alpha-ANP may be atrial compression by the distended lungs and the well-known reduction of venous return to the heart.

2. **Osmoreceptor**

ADH feed-back control mechanism an increase in the osmolality (mainly excess of Na+ CI- or HC03) excites the osmoreceptors located in the anterior hypothalamus-thirst center, which in turn causes release of ADH which is secreted from supraoptic nuclei of posterior pituitary. ADH increases the permeability of DCT & CD to water & therefore causes increased conservation of water, by formation of concentrated urine. Conversely when CF becomes hypo osmotic; less ADH is formed & dilute urine is excreted [51]

3. **Sodium excretion & its control by aldosterone**

When the extracellular fluid (ECF) volume drops significantly, pro-rennin stored in the juxtaglomerular cells is transformed into its active form, renin. Renin then acts on the angiotensinogen in the blood to produce angiotensin I, which has slight vasoconstrictor effects.

With a few seconds angiotensin I is converted to angiotensin II by converting enzymes present in the endothelium of renal vessels. Angiotensin II is a potent vasoconstrictor & causes the adrenal glands to secrete aldosterone; which in turn increases salt & water absorption by renal tubules.[52]

DISTURBANCES IN WATER METABOLISM

a) Pure water depletion

This condition is uncommon in adults but more prevalent in children, who have a less effective ability to concentrate urine. In adults, it can occur in cases of coma or following surgery, where both fluid and electrolyte levels can become depleted.

CAUSES:

- Difficulty/inability to swallow because of. painful conditions of the mouth & pharynx or obstruction in the esophagus
- Increased loss from lungs after tracheostomy. After tracheostomy humidification of the inspired air is an important preventive measure

- Loss from GIT: vomiting, diarrhea, intestinal fistulae,
- Diabetes insipidus
- Coma with inadequate fluid intake
- Sequestration of fluid in infection, burns & soft tissue injuries [3]

PATHOPHYSIOLOGY

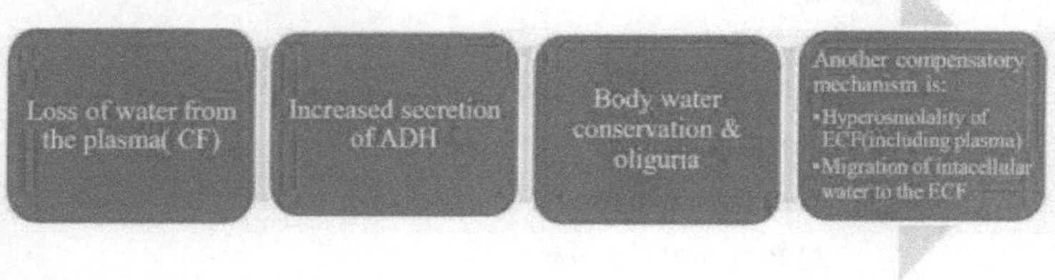

This restores the ECF volume to some extent but causes shrinkage of the ICF.

SIGN & SYMPTOMS

1) **CNS Symptoms**
- Early-thirst, weakness, sleepiness, hypothermia
- Late-decreased reflex
- Stupor
- Coma

2) **CVS Symptoms**
- Hypotension,
- Tachycardia
- Collapsed vein
- Cold extremities
- Thready pulse

3) **GIT**
- Nausea
- Vomiting
- Anorexia

LABORATORY DATA:

1. Specific gravity of urine is high
2. Azotemia (non protein nitrogen high)
3. Elevation of hematocrit
4. Low or absent Na & CI from urine

TREATMENT:

1. Intake of water must be increased initially
2. If not possible I.V dextrose/dextrose saline given
3. Careful chart of intake & output is maintained
4. Care must be taken not to overload & cause water intoxication

b) Pure water excess

The ability of our body to discard extra water being very powerful, pure water intoxication does not occur easily [53]

CAUSES

- Iatrogenic conditions: Excessive administration of I.V fluids
- Pathological conditions:
    - After major surgical operation (it is now known that in addition to cortisol, ADH is also secreted in heavy amounts in conditions of stress)
    - Congestive heart failure
    - Renal failure
    - After the use of some drugs in heavier amount (increase release of ADH by indomethacin, phenylbutazone, carbamazepine falls in this category)

INTERSTITIAL FLUID DYNAMICS

Intrinsic lymphatic pumping is regulated by four major factors- preload, afterload, spontaneous contraction frequency and contractility [3].

Preload is the end-diastolic pressure (or volume) within the valved muscular lymphangion. Increasing the 'filling pressure' over a physiologic range increases the amplitude of contraction and so enhances pump output.

Afterload: The lymphatic pump must adapt to elevated outflow pressures resulting from partial outflow obstruction, increased central venous pressure and/or gravitational shifts. Lymphangion in series can propel lymph against higher pressures than individual lymphangion.

Contraction frequency of collecting lymphatics is exquisitely sensitive to pressure, and changes as small as 0.5 cm H_2O can double the contraction frequency [3].

Contractility is often used in the lymphatic context to describe the enhancement of amplitude or frequency of contraction in response to a pressure increase or agonist activation. The cardiac parallel is the concept of inotropy and inotropic agents.

The 5 Ps of Fluid Prescription

- Prescriber: makes a clinical decision regarding fluid management
- Prescription: is written, accounting for drug, dose and duration
- Pharmacist: checks the prescription for inconsistencies
- Preparation: prescribed fluid is prepared with any necessary additions (e.g. electrolytes)
- Patient: fluid is administered to the patient; the process, response and follow-up management are handled by fluid stewards [3].

II) ELECTROLYTE BALANCE

Both intracellular & extracellular compartments have:

Cations - which are electro positive, e.g. Na, K, Ca, Mg

Anions - which are electro negative, e.g. CI, phosphorous, bicarbonate, sulphate

These are known as electrolytes & the balance between them is known as electrolyte balance. The distribution of these within the fluid compartments of body controls the acid base equilibrium [54]

NORMAL PLASMA CONCENTRATIONS	
SODIUM	135-145 m E g/l
POTASSIUM	3.8-5.5 m E g/l
CHOLORIDE	95-105m E g/l
BICARBONATES	25-30 m E g/l

ELECTROLYTE DISTURBANCES

A) SODIUM

Sodium is the primary cation found outside of cells and plays a key role in regulating the osmolality of extracellular fluid. Around 44% of the body's total protein is located in the extracellular fluid, 9% is within intracellular fluid, and the remaining 47% is stored in the bones. The average daily sodium requirement is approximately 1-2 mEq/kg [55]

Normal blood sodium levels range from 135 to 145 milliequivalents per liter (mEq/L). Hyponatremia is diagnosed when sodium levels drop below 135 mEq/L, while hypernatremia occurs when levels exceed 145 mEq/L. Sodium balance in the body is regulated through multiple mechanisms. Typically, adequate sodium intake is achieved through diet, and the kidneys adjust sodium excretion to maintain proper balance [56]

.

A) HYPERNATREMIA (SODIUM EXCESS)

CAUSES

i) Real causes

- Kidney diseases e.g.: Acute glomerulonephritis where the elimination of sodium by kidney is unsatisfactory.
- Heart failure where a reduction of glomerular filtration rate ultimately leads to sodium accumulation.
- Iatrogenic conditions
- excessive administration of cortisol
- excessive use of normal saline in hospital wards to treat cases of severe diarrhea & in early post operative period as some degree of Na retention occurs [57]

ii) Apparent causes

- Inadequate water intake.
- Hyperventilation

- Diabetes insipidus
- Dehydration

SIGN & SYMPTOMS

- Slight puffiness of face is the only early sign.
- Pitting edema in the sacral region & ankles.
- Patient weight increases & polyuria
- Signs of over hydration in infancy are: increased tension in anterior fontanelle, increases weight, increase in number of urination & edema [58]
- Hypertension, Muscle weakness, restlessness extreme thirst, confusion, lethargy, irritability,
- neurological defects can appear, including ataxia, tremor, coma, and seizures.

PATHOPHYSIOLOGY

Retention of sodium causes

↓

Hyperosmolarity of ECF

↓

Stimulation of ADH secretion

↓

Conservation of water

Thus, sodium accumulation ultimately causes accumulation of both water & sodium. ECF expands. These signs and symptoms are due to ECF expansion.

LABORATORY DATA

Plasma sodium above 145 mEq/L

Specific gravity of urine more than 1.025

TREATMENT

- Sodium input must be restricted & excretion must be increased by giving diuretics.
- Pulmonary edema treated by aminophylline.
- Mild case can be treated by fluid intake but for more serious cases iv line should be used, intravenous fluid choice includes 5% dextrose (most preferred), 0.9% saline (used if evidence of volume depletion) or Hartmann's solution.

B) HYPONATREMIA (SODIUM DEPLETION)

CAUSES

i) Real causes

- Addisons disease where there is lack of aldosterone
- Burns
- Increased loss in sweat.
- Loss from GIT : vomiting , diarrhea, intestinal fistula

ii) Apparent causes

- When replacement is done only with water or glucose & not with ions in particular to sodium ions
- Sodium excretion shut down of trauma [59]:

Decreased renal excretion of sodium is a well-known feature of the immediate postoperative state. The mechanisms responsible have, however, not been clearly defined. While increased adrenal cortical secretion such as is generally associated with major surgical procedures has been causally implicated by many investigators, there is considerable evidence that the changes in sodium excretion are independent of variations in the supply of adrenal cortical hormones. The extracellular fluid volume, or more precisely that portion of it which is physiologically "effective," has been shown to be a major determinant of renal sodium excretion in normal individuals. Therefore, variation in this volume warrants consideration as a possible etiological factor in the decreased postoperative excretion of sodium. The observations that fluid sequestration occurs in and about the traumatized tissues in man indeed suggests that a dislocation of the body fluids may occur in the surgical patient and result in a contraction of the effective extracellular fluid volume.

- Following trauma of any kind there is almost non excretion of sodium for at least 48 hours & due to increased adrenocortical activity. During this period, output of Na cannot be increased by a supplemented intake of sodium. For this reason, it is not advisable to administer large quantities of isotonic 0.9% saline solution after an operation [59].

PATHOPHYSIOLOGY

As the sodium is depleted, the following chain of events develops as compensatory mechanism:

Sodium loss from ECF

⇩

Fall of osmolarity of the ECF

⇩

Stoppage of ADH secretion

⇩

Elimination of large volume of excessively dilute urine

- This causes shrinkage of volume of ECF.

The early signs & symptoms are due to shrinkage of ECF. If the loss of sodium continues further compensatory mechanism are called into action.

Thus

- Fall in osmolarity of the ECF
- Movement of ECF water into inside of the cells
- Swelling of the cells
- Many late stage & symptoms of sodium depletion are due to cellular swelling

SIGNS & SYMPTOMS

1) CNS symptoms:

- Apprehension, hyperactive reflexes,

- confusion.

2) **FACE**:
   - Eyes are sunken;
   - face is drawn with anxious expression.
3) **TONGUE**:
   - Tongue is dry and hard though the patient is not thirsty.
   - Reddish brown in color
4) **SKIN**:
   - The skin is dry, wrinkled
   - the subcutaneous tissue feels laxed.
   - In one word the patient appears to have aged by many years in few hours[60].
5) **B.P**:
   - It reduces & the pulse rate becomes fast.
   - Peripheral veins are poorly filled.
6) **URINE**:
   - It becomes dark & scanty with high specific gravity.
7) In infants the anterior fontanelle is depressed.

LABORATORY DATA

- Plasma level, of sodium is less than 130mEq/L.
- Oligourea, Specific gravity of urine is increased.

TREATMENT

The first step in treatment is to administer normal saline (o.9%) through I.V drip. In the beginning the infusion rate must be rapid to make good sodium concentration [61] Ringer's solution can be used if normal saline is not available. Hypertonic saline should only be used when there is central nervous system symptoms caused by hyponatremia. Renal function needs to be monitored, and it's important to avoid excessive infusion.

Post-operative hyponatremia requires careful fluid balance. Start close fluid monitoring, catheterizing if necessary; this is particularly important during the intraoperative and post-operative period.

Intravenous fluids (such as 0.9% sodium chloride) are generally advised over enteral hydration for the hyponatremic patient, as they will provide a greater control to the serum electrolyte levels. Monitor renal function and electrolyte levels regularly, as potential derangement may occur during any fluid redistribution during your management. If the cause is unknown or evidence of prolonged and marked hyponatremia, urine osmolality and sodium concentration should be measured to inform additional diagnosis.

B) <u>POTASSIUM</u>

This is mainly an intracellular cation (98%). Only 2% is in extracellular fluid. Normal plasma concentration is 3.8-5.5 mEq/L0 The daily requirement is 0.6 mEq/kg/day. Nearly the same amount is excreted in the urine each day, with only a small amount being eliminated through feces and sweat.

A) HYPOKALEMIA (POTASSIUM DEPLETION)

1. Following trauma (which includes operation), there is increased mobilization of intracellular potassium extracellular space & there is increased excretion of potassium by kidneys specially during first day.

   In starvation, as a result of catabolism of protein tissues potassium & nitrogen are excreted in the urine in the same proportion as they are found in the skeletal mass [22]
2. Loss of GIT secretions:
   - Severe vomiting
   - Diarrhoea
   - Aspiration
   - Diseases like diabetes
   - Excessive cortisone or ACTH therapy.

PATHOPHYSIOLOGY

As the body losses potassium, the plasma potassium tends to fall, but K+ of ICF comes to replenish the losses so that, at least in the early stages, plasma K+ levels may be within the normal limits & the K+ deficiency occurs only in ICF23 As the resulting membrane potential on K+, the reduction of K+ concentration in the ICF causes abnormal resting potential & abnormality of excitability & conductivity appear in the muscles & nerves [63]

SIGN & SYMPTOMS

- Gradual onset of drowsiness
- The speech is slurred & slow, fails to complete sentence.
- Reflexes are lost & incontinence of urine.
- Muscular hypotonia & weakness of muscles.
- Decreased B.P & pulse.
- Skin is warm, dry & peripheral veins are well filled
- Patient is thirsty & may drink more quantity of water [61].

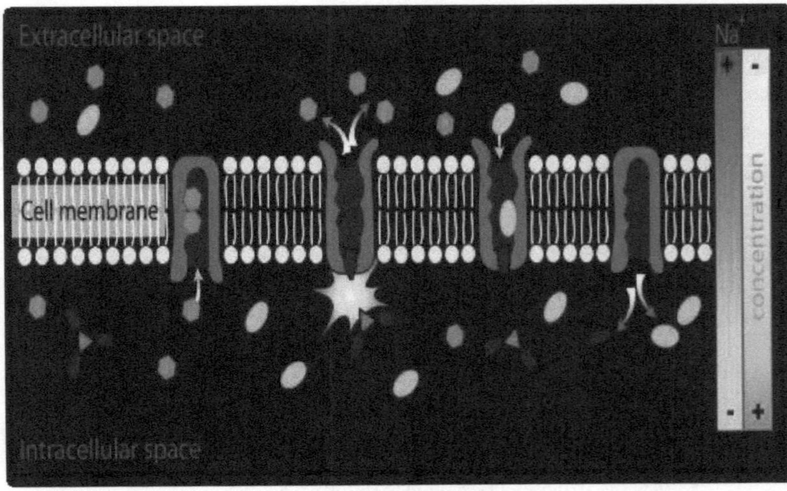

FIGURE 4 - pathophysiology of potassium

Courtesy: Google
https://www.google.com/imgres?q=POTASSIUM%20PATHOPHYSIOLOGY&imgurl=https%3A%2F%2Fwww.wikidoc.org%2Fimages%2F1%2F13%2FHypokalemia_.png&imgrefurl=https%3A%2F%2Fwww.wikidoc.org%2Findex.php%2FHypokalemia_pathophysiology&docid=0Fn2_zpvPbYgfM&tbnid=LjZwny3ZcWgDGM&vet=12ahUKEwikn6Xd1PaIAxWwbmwGHdMHPYUQM3oECE0QAA.i&w=1920&h=833&hcb=2&ved=2ahUKEwikn6Xd1PaIAxWwbmwGHdMHPYUQM3oECE0QAA

LABORATORY DATA

- potassium is less than 3.2 mEg/L.
- polyuria with dilute urine.

MANAGEMENT

Replacement of large deficit of potassium involves the administration of sufficient potassium & its transfer into depleted cells whenever possible.

Potassium salt should be taken orally in the form of effervescent tablets, with doses of 2-6 grams per hour.

Oral potassium is generally preferred to prevent the risk of elevated potassium levels that can occur with intravenous administration of potassium salts in solutions like milk extracts, fruit juices, and honey. However, intravenous administration becomes necessary if the patient is comatose, nauseated, or has difficulty swallowing.

Infusing even a small amount, such as 1 gram of KCL, can sometimes restore consciousness. It's crucial to avoid raising the potassium concentration in the extracellular fluid above 7 mEq/L, as this level is toxic and could lead to cardiac arrest. Before administering potassium intravenously, ensure that urine flow is adequate. Hypokalemia is often linked with alkalosis or occasionally with acidosis. In cases of alkalosis, KCL can be administered intravenously at 2 grams every four hours. For acidosis, a combination of KCL and sodium acetate should be given intravenously [64].

B) HYPERKALEMIA (POTASSIUM EXCESS)

It is mainly iatrogenic & occurs due to excessive I.V administration of potassium salts.

LABORATORY DATA

Plasma' potassium level above 6 m Eq/L

SIGN & SYMPTOMS

- GIT- Nausea, vomiting, intermittent colic & diarrhea
- CVS-Heart rate increase, decrease in B.P, poor peripheral circulation.

MANAGEMENT

Reduction of blood serum potassium level by:

- Potassium intake must be discontinued.
- Temporarily counteract the myocardial effects caused by a sudden increase in potassium concentration, intravenous administration of 10-30 milliliters of 10% calcium gluconate over 15-30 minutes can

- be performed, with ECG monitoring.
- 3. 5% glucose rapid infusion - this stimulates insulin release which helps in cellular uptake of potassium.

C) CALCIUM

Calcium is mainly an extracellular cation & its normal level is between 9-11 mg per 100ml. The normal daily intake of calcium is between 1-3 gm. The majority of calcium is in the bone in the form of phosphate & carbonate [65]

Calcium in the serum is available in the three forms:

- About half is bound to plasma protein
- About 5% of non-ionized fraction is bound to other substances in the plasma & interstitial fluids.
- The remaining 45% of calcium in its ionized form plays a crucial role in neuromuscular stability. Therefore, the ratio of ionized to non-ionized calcium is influenced by plasma protein levels and the ph.

A) HYPOCALCEMIA (CALCIUM EXCESS)

CAUSES

- Acute pancreatitis, massive soft tissue infection
- Inadequate intake
- Or absorption
- vitamin D deficiency
- Hypothyroidism
- Severe Mg depletion

SIGN & SYMPTOMS

Symptoms of hypocalcemia are seen when serum calcium level fall below 8mg/dl. They include:

- Numbness & tingling sensation in the circumoral region & tips of finger & toes

- Hyperactive tendon jerks, muscle cramps with Carpopedal spasms & tetany [66].
- The Chvosteks sign will be positive.

TREATMENT

- I.V administration of calcium gluconate or chloride.
- Calcium lactate may be given orally with supplement of vitamin D

B) **HYPERCALCEMIA**

A serum calcium concentrates above 15 mg/100ml is a serious condition & requires immediate treatment [67].

CAUSES:

- Hyperparathyroidism
- Vitamin D intoxication
- Osteolysis due to metastatic carcinoma,
- Paget's disease, T. B

SIGN & SYMPTOMS

- Anorexia, nausea, vomiting, fatigue & weakness are the main symptoms in the early stage
- With more high serum calcium levels headache, pain in the extremities, thirst, polyuria, stupor & finally coma occurs.

TREATMENT

- Oral & I.V administration of inorganic phosphates effectively lower serum calcium by inhibiting bone resorption & forming calcium phosphates complexes that are deposited in soft tissue & bone
- corticosteroids decrease resorption of calcium from bone. It's useful in treating patients with sarcoidosis, myeloma, lymphoma & leukemia

- calcitonin also decreases serum calcium level
- Mithramycin, a cytotoxic drug lowers serum calcium level in one or two days by direct action on bones.

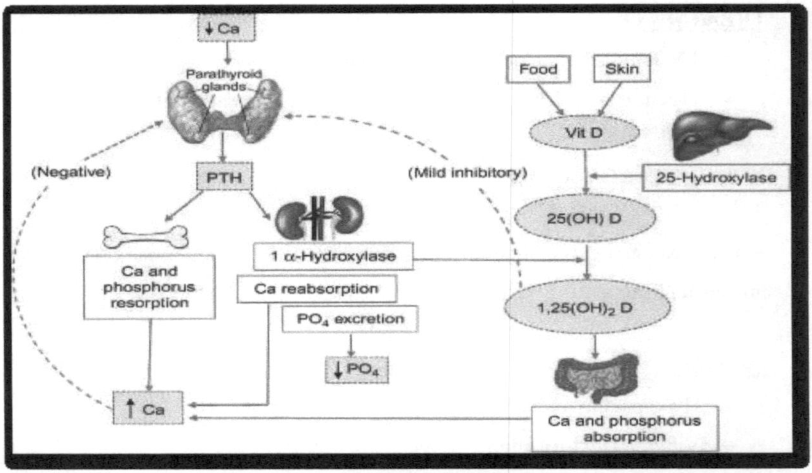

Figure-5 - Calcium metabolism

Courtesy- Song L. Calcium and bone metabolism indices. Advances in clinical chemistry. 2017 Jan 1;82:1-46.

D) MAGNESIUM

Magnesium is an important ion in the maintenance of normal contractility of muscle & excitability of neural tissue. The plasma concentrate of magnesium in normal individual varies between 1.7-2.2 mEq/L[68]. About half of the magnesium is in bone & nearly all the rest is in the cells of soft tissues whereas less than 1% is in extracellular fluid.

A) MAGNESIUM DEFICIENCY

Since ordinary food stuff contain an abundant amount of magnesium, magnesium deficiency is extremely rare in health.

CAUSES

- Reduction in intake, particularly in chronic alcoholics in which excretion of magnesium in the urine is increased by ingestion of alcohol
- Starvation
- Malabsorption syndrome
- Cirrhosis of liver
- Disease of parathyroids

SIGN & SYMPTOMS

- Often accompanies hypocalcemia
- Increased membrane excitability muscle cramps, paraesthesia
- positive Chvosteks & Trosseau sign
- Mental status changes & weakness,
- Arrhythmia, atrial or ventricular fibrillation, widened
- QRS complex, peaked T wave, prolonged P-R & 0-T interval

MANAGEMENT

Magnesium deficiency is best treated by parenteral administration of magnesium chloride or sulphate solution. About 2mEq/L of magnesium per kg body weight may be administered daily when the renal function is good. Magnesium ion should not be given to oliguria patient due to chance of magnesium toxicity [69]

B) MAGNESIUM EXCESS:

- Increase in magnesium ion can occur due to:
- •Excessive intake (iatrogenic, antacids, enema)
- •Inadequate excretion (renal failure, Addison disease, lithium administration due to redistribution of magnesium due to metabolic acidosis)

SIGN & SYMPTOMS

- weakness
- progressive loss of deep tendon reflex
- interference with cardiac conduction & E.C.G changes in the form of increased P-R interval, widened QRS complex & elevated T wave
- gradual muscle paralysis & coma death may occur due to respiratory or cardiac arrest

TREATMENT:

- cessation of magnesium administration syndrome may be controlled by slow administration of 5-10mEg of calcium chloride or gluconate.
- However, for elevated levels & persistence acute symptoms, peritoneal dialysis or hemodialysis should be called for.

E) PHOSPHATE

About 85% of the total phosphate is stored in the bones, with 99% of it being intracellular. This intracellular phosphate is primarily composed of organic phosphates, including phospholipids, nucleic acids, nucleotides, phosphoproteins, and intermediates involved in carbohydrate metabolism.
A small amount of inorganic phosphate in body fluids exists as the anion HPO_4^{2-}. This phosphate is essential for the synthesis of organic phosphates and plays a key role as a buffer in the body [70]

A) PARATHYROID HORMONE (PTH)

Parathyroid hormone (PTH) is a hormone that your parathyroid glands make and release to control the level of calcium in your blood, not your bones. Calcium is one of the most important and common minerals in your body. PTH also helps control the levels of phosphorus (a mineral) and vitamin D (a hormone) in your blood and bones.

Action of Paratharmone

Parathyroid hormone regulates calcium levels in your blood by affecting the following parts of your body:

- Bones: Parathyroid hormone stimulates the release of small amounts of calcium from your bones into your bloodstream.
- Kidneys: Parathyroid hormone enables the production of active vitamin D (calcitriol) in your kidneys. PTH also signals your kidneys to retain calcium in your body rather than flushing it out through your urine.
- Small intestine: Parathyroid hormone signals your small intestine to absorb more calcium from the food you eat.
- It also regulates Mg, decreased Mg causes increased secretion of P

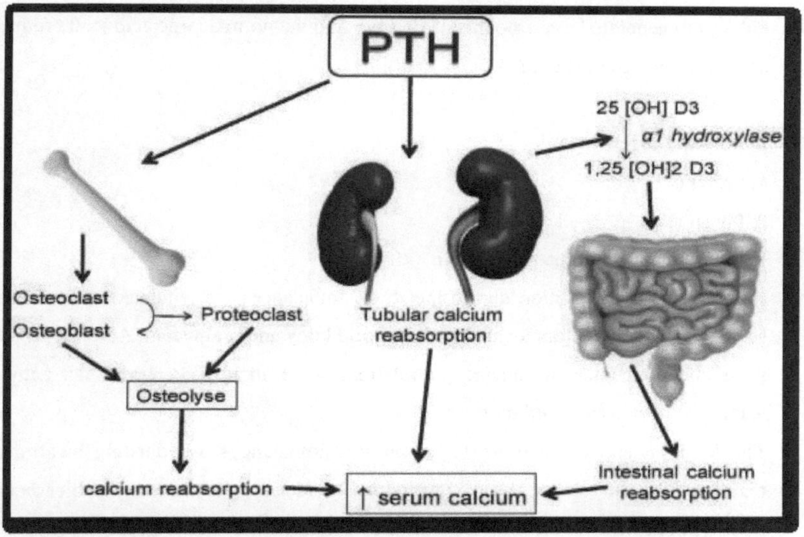

Figure 6- Action of PTH

Courtesy: Casarim AL. Parathyroid Glands and Hyperparathyroidism: A General Overview. Mineral Deficiencies-Electrolyte Disturbances, Genes, Diet and Disease Interface. 2020 Jun 11.

ACID BASE BALANCE

In health the range of pH of blood is 7.36-7.44. the terms alkalosis & acidosis indicate change or tendency to change in the pH of the blood in a particular detection. In acidosis there is accumulation of acid or loss of base causing a fall or tendency to a fall in pH. The converse is true in alkalosis.

Blood pH is regulated by various buffering systems, primarily made up of weak acids or weak bases. The most crucial of these is the bicarbonate-carbonic acid system, represented by the HCO_3^-/H_2CO_3 ratio. Typically, this ratio is 20:1. Any change in this ratio affects the pH level; a decrease in the ratio results in increased acidity, while an increase leads to reduced acidity [71].

The pH of body fluids is maintained within a narrow range despite the ability of the kidneys to generate large amounts of HCO_3- and the normal large acid load produced as a byproduct of metabolism.

Important Buffers Include

1. Proteins
2. Phosphates
3. Bicarbonate–carbonic acid system.

Adjustments in ventilation due to metabolic imbalances are regulated by hydrogen-sensitive chemoreceptors located in the carotid body and brain stem. Acidosis triggers these chemoreceptors to enhance ventilation, while alkalosis reduces their activity, leading to decreased ventilation.

The kidneys help compensate for respiratory imbalances by adjusting bicarbonate reabsorption. In response to respiratory acidosis, they increase bicarbonate reabsorption, while in the case of respiratory alkalosis, they decrease it.

The major acid-base buffering system in the blood involves carbon dioxide and bicarbonate anion.

$$H^+ + HCO_3- \leftrightarrow H_2C0_3 \leftrightarrow CO2 + H_2O$$

The relationship between the species that define pH is known as the Henderson-Hasselbalch Equation:

$$pH = 6.1 + \log HCO_3^- / 0.03 \times PaCo_2$$

a) ACIDOSIS

i) METABOLIC ACIDOSIS

This is a condition in which there is gain or retention of fixed acids or loss of bases. Metabolic acidosis is primary reduction in bicarbonate (HCO_3^-), typically with compensatory reduction in carbon dioxide partial pressure (Pco_2); pH may be markedly low or slightly subnormal. Metabolic acidosis is categorized as high or normal anion gap based on the presence or absence of unmeasured anions in serum. Causes include accumulation of ketones and lactic acid, renal failure, and drug or toxin ingestion (high anion gap) and gastrointestinal or renal $HCO3^-$ loss (normal anion gap). Symptoms and signs in severe cases include nausea and vomiting, lethargy, and hyperpnea. Diagnosis is clinical and with arterial blood gas (ABG) and serum electrolyte measurement. The cause is treated; IV sodium bicarbonate may be indicated when pH is very low [71].

CAUSES

1) Gain of fixed acids may occur:
    - Due to formation of ketone bodies as in diabetes or starvation
    - The retention of metabolites in renal insufficiency
    - Rapid increase in lactic acid & purvic acids by anaerobic tissue metabolism due to shock
    - Rapid blood transfusion done with blood bank containing citrate
2) Loss of such bases may occur in:
    - Sustained diarrhea
    - Ulcerative colitis,

- Git fistulae,
- High intestinal fistula

CLINICAL FEATURES:

- Most marked clinical sign is rapid, deep & noisy respirations which is often called air hunger (kassumal breathing)
- Patient also tries unsuccessfully to moisten his lips with his parched tongue.
- Excessive breathing expels carbonic acid as co2. Additionally, the kidneys work to counteract acidosis by conserving sodium, which helps to elevate the ph.
- The urine becomes strongly acidic.
- The pulse rate & the blood pressure may be also raised.

TREATMENT

- If causes are due to gain of acids then slow infusion of dilute sodium bicarbonate solution should be given. Initial dose should not exceed 50ml of 7.5% solution.
- If there are other causes then sodium bicarbonate infusion along with R.L solution should be given.
- Treatment of acidemia with sodium bicarbonate ($NaHCO_3$) is clearly indicated only in certain circumstances and is probably deleterious in others. When metabolic acidosisresults from loss of HCO_3^- or accumulation of inorganic acids (ie, normal anion gap acidosis), bicarbonate therapy is generally safe and appropriate. However, when acidosis results from organic acid accumulation (ie, high anion gap acidosis), bicarbonate therapy is controversial; it does not clearly decrease mortality in these conditions, and there are several possible risks.
- With treatment of the underlying condition, lactate and ketoacids are metabolized back to HCO_3^-; exogenous HCO_3^- loading may therefore cause an "overshoot" metabolic alkalosis.

ii) RESPIRATORY ACIDOSIS

Respiratory acidosis is primary increase in carbon dioxide partial pressure (Pco2) with or without compensatory increase in bicarbonate (HCO_3^-); pH is usually low but may be near normal. Cause is a decrease in respiratory rate and/or volume (hypoventilation), typically due to central nervous system, pulmonary, or iatrogenic conditions. Respiratory acidosis can be acute or chronic; the chronic form is asymptomatic, but the acute, or worsening, form causes headache, confusion, and drowsiness. Signs include tremor, myoclonic jerks, and asterixis. Diagnosis is clinical and with arterial blood gas and serum electrolyte measurements.

The cause is treated; oxygen (O_2) and mechanical ventilation are often required [2].

This is less common than metabolic type.

CAUSES

- When there is inadequate ventilation
- When in an ansesthesized patient the effect of muscle relaxants have not worn off.
- Certain lung disorders
- Emphysema,
- Chronic
- Bronchitis, bronchopneumonia
- Crushing or other injuries of chest
- Respiratory center may be depressed by brain injury or by poisoning with alcohol, barbiturate drugs morphine
- airway obstruction

CLINICAL FEATURES:

- Restlessness,
- Hypertension,
- Tachycardia.

TREATMENT:

Immediate treatment should ensure adequate ventilation by endotracheal intubation & mechanical ventilation & over use of muscle relaxants must be avoided. Treatment is provision of adequate ventilation by either endotracheal intubation or non-invasive positive pressure ventilation. Adequate ventilation is all that is needed to correct respiratory acidosis. Chronic hypercapnia generally must be corrected slowly (e.g., over several hours or more) because too-rapid Pco2 lowering can cause a post hypercapnic "overshoot" alkalosis when the underlying compensatory hyperbicarbonatemia becomes unmasked. The abrupt rise in CNS pH that results can lead to seizures and death. Any potassium and chloride deficits are corrected.

Sodium bicarbonate is almost always contraindicated because of the potential for paradoxical acidosis within the CNS.

B) ALKALOSIS

i) METABOLIC ALKALOSIS:

Metabolic alkalosis is primary increase in bicarbonate (HCO_3^-) with or without compensatory increase in carbon dioxide partial pressure (Pco2); pH may be high or nearly normal. Common causes include prolonged vomiting, hypovolemia, diuretic use, and hypokalemia. Renal impairment of HCO_3^- excretion must be present to sustain alkalosis. Symptoms and signs in severe cases include headache, lethargy, and tetany. Diagnosis is clinical and with arterial blood gas and serum electrolyte measurement. The underlying condition is treated; oral or IV acetazolamide or hydrochloric acid is sometimes indicated.

CAUSES

- Excessive ingestion of absorbable alkali. Common in patients taking various antacids or ingestion remedies without medical supervision
- Loss of acid from the stomach is repeated by vomiting or aspiration
- prolonged administration of Cortisone, ACTH [72]

- To compensate for alkalosis there is:
- retention. Of CO_2 by lungs, which combine with water to form carbonic acid
- excretion of bicarbonate base by kidneys (alkaline urine)

CLINICAL FEATURES

Mild degree of alkalosis does not cause particular clinical features in severe cases the most striking feature of the alkalosis is the phasic respiration, which is a period of apnea of 30 seconds or maximum followed by onset of respiration which at first is shallow & then increases in depth until the expiration is normal [73]. After 2-3 normal respirations of normal range & it again declines to aponia. Tetany may occur in severe alkalosis due to combination of free Ca ions.

This is the cause of increased irritability of skeletal muscles.

Latent tetanus is more common which is revealed by Trousseaus sign.

TREATMENT

- To remove the cause
- Maintain an adequate volume of blood
- Bring down alkalosis by giving ammonium chloride
- Potassium depletion goes in hand in hand with metabolic alkalosis so i.v infusion of a solution of potassium chloride is also necessary
- IV 0.9% saline solution for chloride-responsive metabolic alkalosis
- Underlying conditions are treated, with particular attention paid to correction of hypovolemia and hypokalemia.
- Patients with chloride-responsive metabolic alkalosis are given 0.9% saline solution IV; infusion rate is typically 50 to 100 ml/hour greater than urinary and other sensible and insensible fluid losses until urinary cl rises to > 25 meq/l (> 25 mmol/l) and urinary ph normalizes after an initial rise from bicarbonaturia.

ii) **RESPIRATORY ALKALOSIS**:

Respiratory alkalosis is a condition in which the carbon dioxide tension in arterial blood is below normal range. Respiratory alkalosis occurs when low carbon dioxide levels disrupt your blood's acid-base balance. It often occurs in people who experience rapid, uncontrollable breathing (hyperventilation). Treatment includes supplemental oxygen and therapies to reduce the risk of hyperventilation

CAUSES

- During anesthesia
- Excessive pulmonary
- Ventilation is carried out without use of muscle relaxant
- May also occur due to apprehension, pain or CNS injury due to hysteria
- In men at high altitudes & those working in very dry atmosphere
- High fever, salicylate or carbon monoxide poisoning
- Compensation depends on the increased renal excretion of bicarbonate

CLINICAL FEATURES

- Pallor, fall in B.P. in severe cases respiratory arrest might follow breathlessness.
- Numbness and /or tingling in your fingertips, toes and lips.
- Irritability, Nausea, Dizziness.
- Muscle spasms or twitching, Fatigue., Dizziness/light-headedness. Fainting (syncope).
- Chest discomfort, Shortness of breath, tremors, Confusion.

TREATMENT

Respiratory arrest due to alkalosis is immediately corrected by in suffusion of CO_2. Potassium deficit is corrected by giving KCI because in alkalosis as compensatory measure K ion is lost along with HCO_3 ion.

FLUID AND ELECTROLYTE REGULATION

The body must carefully regulate intravascular fluid accumulation and excretion to prevent fluid volume excesses or deficits and maintain adequate blood pressure. Water balance is regulated by several mechanisms including ADH, thirst, and the Renin-Angiotensin-Aldosterone System (RAAS) [1].

Fluid intake is regulated by thirst. Serum **osmolality** is a measure of the concentration of dissolved solutes in the blood. Osmoreceptors in the hypothalamus sense increased serum osmolarity levels and trigger the release of ADH (antidiuretic hormone) in the kidneys to retain fluid.

They must be alert, fluids must be accessible, and the person must be strong enough to reach for fluids. When a person is unable to respond to thirst signals, dehydration occurs. Older individuals are at increased risk of dehydration due to age-related impairment in thirst perception. The average adult intake of fluids is about 2,500 mL per day from both food and drink. An increased number of fluids is needed if the patient has other medical conditions causing excessive fluid loss, such as sweating, fever, vomiting, diarrhea, and bleeding [1].

The **Renin-Angiotensin-Aldosterone System (RAAS)** plays an important role in regulating fluid output and blood pressure. When there is decreased blood pressure (which can be caused by fluid loss), specialized kidney cells make and secrete renin into the bloodstream. Renin acts on angiotensinogen released by the liver and converts it to angiotensin I, which is then converted to angiotensin II. Angiotensin II does a few important things. First, angiotensin II causes vasoconstriction to increase blood flow to vital organs. It also stimulates the adrenal cortex to release aldosterone. Aldosterone is a steroid hormone that triggers increased sodium reabsorption by the kidneys and subsequent increased serum osmolality in the bloodstream. As you recall, increased serum osmolality causes osmosis to move fluid into the intravascular compartment in an effort to equalize solute particles. The increased fluids in the intravascular compartment increase circulating blood volume and help raise the person's blood pressure. An easy way to remember this physiological process is "aldosterone saves salt" and "water follows salt."

Most fluid output occurs through the kidneys as urine. Additional fluid loss happens through the skin via perspiration, the gastrointestinal tract through stool, and the lungs during breathing. Approximately 40% of daily fluid loss comes from these "insensible losses," which occur through the skin, gastrointestinal tract, and lungs and cannot be precisely measured. The remaining 60% of fluid output is in the form of urine. Typically, the kidneys produce about 1,500 mL of urine daily when fluid intake is sufficient. Reduced urine production can indicate early signs of dehydration or kidney issues. Nurses should monitor urine output closely in at-risk patients. If a patient produces less than 30 mL/hour (or 0.5 mL/kg/hour) of urine over eight hours, the healthcare provider should be informed for timely intervention.

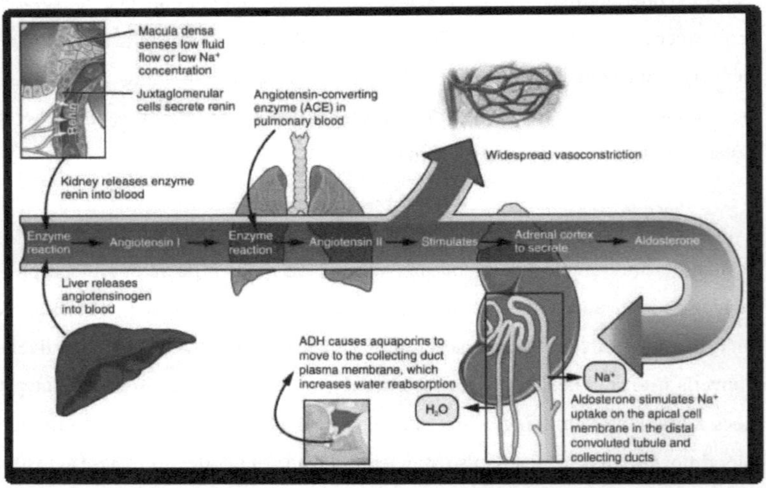

Figure -7 Renin-Angiotensin-Aldosterone System

Courtesy: Open Resources for Nursing (Open RN); Ernst Meyer K, Christman E, editors. Nursing Fundamentals [Internet]. Eau Claire (WI): Chippewa Valley Technical College; 2021. Chapter 15 Fluids and Electrolytes

REPLACEMENTS

SOLUTIONS

1. ***Dextrose 5% solution***

- It is an isotonic solution, which supplies calories but not electrolytes
- It is useful mainly in the very early P.O period when sodium concentration is reduced
- Prolonged administration of 5% dextrose solution is liable to result in - hyponatremia, may cause thrombosis of vein.[74]

2. ***Isotonic (o.9%) sodium chloride saline solution***

It is needed in following conditions –

- When large amount of sodium is lost by vomiting, or by gastric or duodenal or intestinal aspiration or through alimentary fistulae
- This solution is isotonic & contains sodium & chloride in the concentration is 154mEq/L
- One thing to be noticed is that it has concentration of chloride more than plasma concentration (CI 100mEq/L). so, it imposes an appreciable load of excess chloride on the kidney that cannot be readily excreted. Thus, a dilutional acidosis may develop
- This solution is ideal to use in extra cellular fluid deficiency the presence of hyponatremia, hypochloremia, metabolic alkalosis.

FLUID AND ELECTROLYTE THERAPY	Electrolyte Composition (mEq/L)						
Solution	Na	Cl	K	Hco3-	Ca	Mg	mOsm
Extracellular fluid	142	103	4	27	5	3	280-310
Lactated ringers	130	109	4	28	3		273
0.9%sodium chloride	154	154					308
D5 0.45% sodium chloride	77	77					407
D5W							253
3% Sodium chloride	513	513					1026

3. ***Ringer's Lactate solution***

- It contains sodium, potassium, chloride in almost the same concentration as they are in plasma It also contains some calcium & some lactate. This solution is the best to be used in hypovolemic shock while waiting for blood.

- Advantage-
    - It has almost similar concentration as ECF therefore Ph remains normal even after infusion of large quantities.

Disadvantage-

- It has slight hypoosomolarity with respect to sodium
- The transfused blood will coagulate if it is run through an I.V line containing R.L solution. The Ca in lactated R.L negates the anticoagulant effect of citrate in the stored blood. Normal saline should be flushed through the line before any stored blood is administered.

4. ***Dextrose 4.3% with saline 0.18% (one fifth normal saline)***

- This solution is isotonic. Usually, it is referred to as dextrose saline. It must not be confused with 5%dextrose in saline which is hypertonic.
- It can be used in any case of hypovolemia, where there is not considerable depletion of Na & CI
- It has an additional effect of some caloric value.
- It may be infused for prolonged period without any fear of hypernatremia or hyperchloremia [75]. There may be chance of introducing thrombosis.

5. ***Molar (M) sodium lactate solution***

- This solution has a sodium concentration of 1000mEg/L Its anion is lactate instead of chloride
- Uses: this solution is particularly suitable for symptomatic hyponatremia stages and also suitable in metabolic acidosis case.

6. ***Darrow's solution***

- This is only solution which contains more potassium than available in the plasma.

- This is best solution to combat hypokalemia.
- It is safe & convenient method of supplying potassium provided alkalosis is not present.
- Two thumb rules should be applied while prescribing parenteral therapy:

  I) For most of the problems, half of the calculated deficit should be replaced in first 24hours period, with subsequent reassessment of clinical situation

  II) Fluid or electrolyte abnormality should take as long as to correct as it took to develop by adherence to these guidelines overly vigorous replacement will be avoided & along with-it production of different electrolytes abnormality [54]

Four things are considered in balance of fluid electrolytes:

a. Maintenance
b. Fluid Selection
c. Requirement
d. Rate Of Administration

1) MAINTAINANCE

Deficit: mainly volume deficiency is important in this.
This is judged by weight loss of the patient.
On going loss: mainly obligatory loss of both sensible & insensible

2) FLUID SELECTION

• Colloids or crystalloids:
where intravascular loss has occurred earlier are preferred & when extravascular then later is preferred.
Colloids such as blood, albumin
Crystalloids such as dextrose- saline, ringer lactate [2]

	Crystalloid	Colloid
Intravascular persistence	Poor	Good
Haemodynamic stabilization	Transient	Prolonged
Required infusion volume	Large	Moderate
Risk of tissue odema	Obvious	Insignificant
Enhancement of capillary perfusion	Poor	Good
Risk of anaphylaxis	Nill	Low to moderate
Plasma colloid osmotic pressure	Reduced	Maintained
Cost	Inexpensive	Expensive

3) REQUIREMENT

Total loss (deficit + ongoing) +maintenance

Normal requirement: 1500ml for first 20 kg + 20ml/kg body weight/day

4) RATE OF ADMINISTRATION

In children the following formula is used to determine the hourly infusion rate:

- For first 10 kg of B. W: administer 4ml/kg
- For second 10 kg B. W: administer 2 ml/kg
- For each additional kilogram of B.W: administer 1ml/kg

For a 70 kg male, using this formula would result in a rate of 110ml/hr.

- First 10 kg: 10*4=40 ml/hr.
- Second 10 kg: 10*2=20ml/hr.
- Each additional kilogram (70-20) =50kg:50*1=50ml/hr.

Success of fluid & electrolyte can be assessed in following points:

- Increase in B.P
- Decrease in pulse rate
- CVP increases • Serum Na, K, CI, HCO_3 measurements
- pH of blood

• Conditions where P.O fluid & electrolyte measurements is mandatory every 24hr are as follows:

- Sepsis
- preexisting abnormality
- Burns
- extra fluid loss like vomiting, diarrhea
- extensive surgery for 4-6 hours or more

Care should be taken when supplying K during immediate P.O period, because traumatized tissue provides a K load released from injured cells, therefore it is usually unnecessary to give any K supplement in the first 24hr post operatively [76]

REGIME

POST OPERATIVE FLUID REGIME (maintenance)

Most important is to determine volume deficit. In trauma patients, vital signs are normal due to adrenergic compensatory mechanism.

When G.A is given to such patients without adequate replacement of fluid, diastolic hypertension, tachycardia which is followed by hypotension & other problems occur.

This is done by 2 methods:

- measurement of weight loss as it is considered equal to volume loss
- administering chlorpromazine 0.2mg/kg I.V 25% drop in systolic B.P indicates hypovolemia. In normal persons, B.P is not altered.

INTRAOPERATIVE FLUID REGIME:

Intraoperative fluid needs are assessed by monitoring urine output, which should be at least 30 ml per hour or 60% of the administered fluid should be excreted each hour. Additionally, any blood lost during the surgery should be replaced.

POSTOPERATIVE FLUID REGIME:

For minor surgery in which the patient will be able to consume fluids immediately after surgery, fluid deficit is not a major concern. For patients who cannot resume oral intake or has diminished intake during the post operative period, it is important to hydrate the patient. Even for a dent alveolar surgery, however, patients who have been hydrated report feeling better during the immediate post operative period.

PERIOPERATIVE FLUID MANAGEMENT

The outcome after any surgery is dependent on multiple factors among which fluid regulation is an important consideration. The type, amount and rate of fluid administration are primarily determined by the nature of surgery, requirements and losses and coexisting morbidities, if present. Any fluid either too much too little can be of unfavorable consequenses.[3]

Based upon the patient's requirements, fluids can be of either replacement or maintenance type.

1) *Replacement fluids*- During the perioperative period, it is essential to use replacement fluids to address existing deficits or to make up for ongoing losses. Commonly used replacement fluids in this period include 0.9% sodium chloride (NaCl), Ringer's lactate, balanced salt solutions, and synthetic colloids.
2) *Maintenance fluids*- Maintenance fluids are essential for optimizing ongoing losses from physiological processes to maintain homeostasis. Common maintenance fluids include dextrose, dextrose-saline (5% dextrose in 0.9% NaCl), dextrose-hypotonic saline (5% dextrose in 0.45% NaCl), and Isolyte solutions.

The primary goal of preoperative fluid management is to avoid the dehydration of patients before the procedure begins. Clearly, if the patient begins operations in a normal euvolemic condition, it is simpler to maintain an approach of zero balance intraoperatively. Ultimately though, goal-oriented treatment has shown to be a safe operation repeatedly. Better fluid management via improved recovery routes or goals was both proven to decrease postoperative complications on an independent basis. An target based fluid strategy may also provide additional benefit to improved recovery procedures, especially in patients at greater risk, but a large, high-performance clinical study is need to respond conclusively.[77]

CALCULATION OF THIRD-SPACE LOSS

The loss occurring due to fluid shift from the intravascular to the extravascular compartment during surgery is known as third-space loss. This third-space loss follows oedema at the operative site and evaporation from surgical exposure.[3]

The simplest calculation is based upon the type of surgery:

(a) 4 mL/kg/h. for minor and moderate operations (e.g. hernia, hydrocele, cholecystectomy, plating and screwing for limb fractures)

(b) 8 mL/kg/h. for major and supra-major operations (e.g. abdominal hysterectomy,

Whipple's procedure, craniotomy)

(c) The calculation may be also based on the amount of tissue handling or trauma during surgery as suggested in the following table-

Amount of tissue handling or trauma	Fluid requirement (mL/kg/h)
Mild (hernia repair/ophthalmic/otolaryngology procedures)	0–2
Moderate tissue handling (laparoscopic/gynaecologic/ orthopaedic/neurosurgical procedures)	2–4
Major tissue handling (open abdominal surgery, e.g. bowel resection anastomosis)	4–8

Table: Calculation of surgical third space loss based on tissue handling and/or trauma

The fluid challenge remains one of the most essential instruments for an aesthetician to evaluate the fluid response. If the patient is fluid depletion and tolerable for additional fluids, a slim but fast fluid bolus should raise preload enough to produce a detectable rise in the volume of a stroke and in cardiac output.[77]

The UK Enhanced Recovery Consensus statement specifically recommends the use of intraoperative fluid management technology (such as the esophageal Doppler) in any operation, with any of the following features[77].-.

- Major surgery with a 30-day mortality rate of >1 %
- Major surgery with anticipated blood loss of >500 ml
- Major intra-abdominal surgery
- Intermediate surgery (30-day mortality >0.5 %) in high-risk patients (e.g., age > 80, history of left ventricular failure or previous ischemic heart disease or stroke)
- Unexpected blood loss requiring >2 l of fl uid replacement
- Patients with evidence of ongoing hypovolemia or tissue hypoperfusion (e.g., persistent lactic acidosis)

CHOOSING BETWEEN CRYSTALLOIDS AND COLLOIDS

Choosing which intravenous fluid to use is also vitally important to a successful enhanced recovery pathway. Extracellular fluid (ECF) replacement is better replenished by crystalloids. The distribution of crystalloids in the extracellular (interstitial) space is theoretically three times that of the intravascular space. A good option in perioperative patients is to administer the maximum amount of fluid as crystalloids until there is any risk of overload [3].

Insensible losses (such as through perspiration and respiration) should be replaced with balanced crystalloid solutions, and 0.9 % saline solutions (including some colloids that are mixed with 0.9 % solutions) should be avoided wherever possible.[37].

The British Consensus Guidelines on Intravenous Fluid Therapy for Adult Surgical Patients (GIFTASUP) advise that patients receive the following to meet their minimum daily maintenance requirements.

- 1–2 mmol/kg of sodium
- 1 mmol/kg of potassium
- 30 ml/kg water

In terms of replacing other volume losses, most goal-directed fluid studies have used colloid boluses. This is because colloid boluses are thought to increase stroke volume and blood pressure more (and also more quickly) than the same volume of a crystalloid solution, due to colloids being less likely to leak across the glycocalyx and out of intravascular space as rapidly as crystalloid solution [35]

RECOMMENDATIONS FOR PERIOPERATIVE FLUID THERAPY IN MAJOR SURGERY [30]

1. Minimize preoperative fasting times. Encourage unrestricted intake of clear fluids until 2 h before elective surgery.
2. Passive leg raising followed by measurement of blood pressure or (ideally) stroke volume is a useful test for predicting fluid responsiveness in hemodynamically unstable adults throughout the perioperative period.

3. Aim for a moderately liberal IV fluid regimen with an overall positive fluid balance of 1–2 l at the end of surgery. For major abdominal surgery, an average crystalloid fluid infusion rate of 10–12ml · kg−1 · h−1 during surgery, and 1.5ml · kg−1 · h−1 in the 24-h postoperative period should be used.
4. Ensure that intravascular volume status is optimized before adding vasopressor therapy.
5. Use an advanced hemodynamic monitor to measure fluid responsiveness in higher-risk patients having major surgery.
6. A goal-directed hemodynamic strategy may perform better if a patient's IV fluid status is first optimized, and if needed, introduce a vasopressor or inotrope.
7. It is unclear whether crystalloid or colloid should be primarily used for perioperative fluid resuscitation.
8. Aim for early transition from IV to oral fluid therapy after surgery (usually within 24 h).

IV FLUID THERAPY IN NEUROLOGICAL INJURY

In neurologic injury it is best to avoid hypotonic fluids e.g. 5% dextrose or ringer lactate (as it contains 3mEg/L of Ca which promotes reperfusion injury). In head injury its best to use normal saline especially with respect to plasma & it does not contain Ca.

IV FLUID THERAPY IN PEDIATRIC PATIENTS

Fluid resuscitation begins with rapid infusion of 20 ml/kg of crystalloid or colloid

- Access CVS response
- Again 20ml/kg I.V is given
- Access CVS response
- Transfuse packed RBC

IV FLUID THERAPY IN TRAUMATIC HAEMORRHAGIC SHOCK PATIENTS

- Infusion of isotonic crystalloid fluid such as Ringer's Lactate will restore the hemodynamic stability in patients with mild to moderate blood loss.

IV FLUID THERAPY IN BURN PATIENTS

$\%\ of\ body\ surface\ area\ burnt$ × kg weight×4 ml=to amount of fluid required in first 24 hours

Ringer's Lactate Ringer Formula

Transfusion with dextran or plasma is given. All adults with burns over 15% & children with burn over 10% require I.V fluids.

I.V fluids are given after doing a venesection Volume to be transfused-six equal rations of dextran or plasma in six periods is given as follows:

- One ration (in ml) = total % of burns × weight kg)/2
- Three rations are given in first 12 hours
- Two rations are given in the second 12 hours
- One ration is given in the third 12 hours

e.g. in 80 kg weight with 30% burn requires: one ration=80 × 30/2=1200ml

3 × 1200= 3600ml are given in the first 12 hours

2 × 1200= 2400m| are given in the second 12 hour

1 × 1200= 1200ml is given in the next 12hour

I.V dextrose is given for nutritional requirements

FLUID AND ELECTROLYTES RESTORATION

MANAGEMENT OF FLUIDS & ELECTROLYTE

Patients who are undergoing surgery, are ill, or unable to eat due to fasting need to have their fluid and electrolyte balance maintained through parenteral methods. Proper fluid management is essential in medical settings, as each patient has unique needs. While there is no single universal guideline for fluid management, the basic principle of replenishing lost fluids when a deficit is identified applies to all patients. The volume and type of fluid losses can differ based on the patient's medical condition. For example, a patient with severe burns will lose more fluids compared to a generally healthy patient who is fasting before a procedure. Similarly, a patient admitted for dehydration from severe diarrhea might need different fluids than one experiencing hypovolemic shock from a significant upper gastrointestinal bleed.

When administering intravenous (IV) fluids, it is crucial to consider their potential impact on the patient. Each fluid has a distinct composition with varying solutes, possibly leading to metabolic changes.

GOAL OF FLUID MANAGEMENT

- Prevent dehydration
- Prevent electrolyte disorders
- Prevent ketoacidosis
- Prevent protein degradation

PARENTRAL FLUID THERAPY

Methods of administration of fluids:

♣ I. V transfusion

♣ Subcutaneous with hyalase (1000 units of hyaluronidase is mixed with a liter of fluids)

♣ Marrow infusion into tibia

♣ Rectal infusion

♣ Trans nasal intra gastric drip

Rate of flow:

Using plastic transfusion set 15 drops of fluid are approximately equal to 1 ml. At a rate of 30 drops/min/liter solution can be given in 8 hours. In severely dehydrated patients, the rate of I" hour can be accelerated to well over 100 drops per minute after which it should be cut to 50-60 drops[62]. The maintenance dose rate is about 30 drops (3 liters in 24 hours).

CHOICE OF IV FLUID SOLUTIONS

The choice of IV fluid depends on the type of body fluid lost and any associated electrolyte or acid-base abnormalities. The most commonly used fluids in the medical settings are:

- Sodium chloride (0.9%) or normal saline, with or without potassium
- Sodium chloride (0.45%) or half normal saline, with or without potassium
- Lactated Ringer solution
- Dextrose (5%) in sodium chloride (0.9%), with or without potassium.

CONCLUSION

Fluid and electrolyte balance is a crucial aspect of oral surgery, as it can significantly impact a patient's overall health and recovery. Oral surgery procedures can lead to fluid and electrolyte imbalances due to various factors such as bleeding, vomiting, and reduced oral intake. Fluid balance refers to the amount of water and electrolytes in the body, which is regulated by the kidneys, hormones like antidiuretic hormone, aldosterone, RAAS, and other mechanisms like the thirst mechanism.

Maintaining proper fluid balance is essential for regulating body temperature, supporting organ function, and facilitating nutrient transport. Imbalances can lead to dehydration or fluid overload, both of which can cause serious health issues. Electrolytes are minerals such as sodium, potassium, and calcium that help regulate fluid balance and nerve and muscle function. During oral surgery, patients may experience fluid loss due to bleeding or reduced oral intake due to pain or swelling which can lead to dehydration and electrolyte imbalances, and it can cause symptoms such as weakness, dizziness, confusion, and irregular heart rhythms. To maintain fluid and electrolyte balance during oral surgery, patients may receive intravenous fluids and electrolytes to replace any losses. Patients may also be advised to drink plenty of fluids after surgery and consume electrolyte-rich foods such as bananas, yogurt, and sports drinks. After surgery, patients may be encouraged to drink plenty of water and consume electrolyte-rich beverages or supplements to restore their body's balance of minerals such as sodium, potassium, and magnesium. Proper fluid and electrolyte therapy can help to prevent complications such as dehydration, electrolyte imbalances, and postoperative fatigue[80].

It is important for oral surgeons to closely monitor their patients' fluid and electrolyte levels and provide appropriate therapy as needed to support their recovery and overall well-being.[58] Overall, maintaining proper fluid and electrolyte balance is crucial in ensuring successful oral surgery outcomes. Patients should follow their surgeon's instructions carefully and report any symptoms of dehydration or electrolyte imbalances promptly to prevent complications [8]

BIBLIOGRAPHY

1) Open Resources for Nursing (Open RN); Ernst Meyer K, Christman E, editors. Nursing Fundamentals [Internet]. Eau Claire (WI): Chippewa Valley Technical College; 2021. Chapter 15 Fluids and Electrolytes
2) Bailey H, Love R. Chapter 20: Nutrition and fluid therapy. In: Bailey H, Love R, editors. Bailey and Love's Short Practice of Surgery. 26th ed. London: Hodder Arnold; 2013. p. [261-271]
3) Bamboat ZM, Bordeianou L. Perioperative fluid management. Clinics in colon and rectal surgery. 2009 Feb;22(01):028-33.
4) Malbrain ML, Marik PE, Witters I, Cordemans C, Kirkpatrick AW, Roberts DJ, Van Regenmortel N. Fluid overload, de-resuscitation, and outcomes in critically ill or injured patients: a systematic review with suggestions for clinical practice. Anaesthesiol Intensive Ther. 2014;46(5):361–80
5) Jenkins MT, Giesecke AH, Johnson ER. The postoperative patient and his fluid and electrolyte requirements. British Journal of Anaesthesia. 1975 Feb 1;47(2):143-50.
6) Polderman KH, Girbes AR. Severe electrolyte disorders following cardiac surgery: a prospective controlled observational study. Crit Care. 2004;8(6): R459-66.
7) Kraft MD, Btaiche IF, Sacks GS, Kudsk KA. Treatment of electrolyte disorders in adult patients in the intensive care unit. Am J Health Syst Pharm. 2005;62(16):1663-82
8) Hahn RG, Van Regenmortel N. Is the NICE Guideline for Maintenance Fluid Therapy in Adults in Hospital appropriate? Clinical Nutrition ESPEN. 2024 Jun 19.
9) Shires T, Williams J, Brown F. Acute change in extracellular fluids associated with major surgical procedures. Annals of surgery. 1961 Nov 1;154(5):803-10.

10) Virtue RW, LeVine DS, Aikawa JK. Fluid shifts during the surgical period: RISA and S: 35: determinations following glucose, saline or lactate infusion. Annals of Surgery. 1966 Apr 1;163(4):523-8.

11) Mackenzie AI, Donald JR. Urine output and fluid therapy during anaesthesia and surgery. Br Med J. 1969 Sep 13;3(5671):619-22.

12) Jenkins MT, Giesecke AH, Johnson ER. The postoperative patient and his fluid and electrolyte requirements. British Journal of Anaesthesia. 1975 Feb 1;47(2):143-50.

13) Brandstrup B, Tønnesen H, Beier-Holgersen R, Hjortsø E, Ørding H, Lindorff-Larsen K, Rasmussen MS, Lanng C, Wallin L, Iversen LH, Gramkow CS. Effects of intravenous fluid restriction on postoperative complications: comparison of two perioperative fluid regimens: a randomized assessor-blinded multicenter trial. Annals of surgery. 2003 Nov 1;238(5):641-8.

14) Jacka MJ, Alberton D, Noel Gibney RT. Best evidence in critical care medicine: Fluid resuscitation among the critically ill: more water under the bridge. Canadian Journal of Anesthesia. 2006 Dec; 53:1258-9.

15) SAFE Study Investigators. A comparison of albumin and saline for fluid resuscitation in the intensive care unit. New England Journal of Medicine. 2004 May 27;350(22):2247-56.

16) Maharaj CH, Kallam SR, Malik A, Hassett P, Grady D, Laffey JG. Preoperative intravenous fluid therapy decreases postoperative nausea and pain in high-risk patients. Anesthesia & Analgesia. 2005 Mar 1;100(3):675-82.

17) Kabon B, Akça O, Taguchi A, Nagele A, Jebadurai R, Arkilic CF, Sharma N, Ahluwalia A, Galandiuk S, Fleshman J, Sessler DI. Supplemental intravenous crystalloid administration does not reduce the risk of surgical wound infection. Anesthesia & Analgesia. 2005 Nov 1;101(5):1546-53.

18) Lobo DN, Macafee DA, Allison SP. How perioperative fluid balance influences postoperative outcomes. Best practice & research Clinical anaesthesiology. 2006 Sep 1;20(3):439-55.

19) Chappell D, Jacob M, Hofmann-Kiefer K, Conzen P, Rehm M. A rational approach to perioperative fluid management. The Journal of the American Society of Anesthesiologists. 2008 Oct 1;109(4):723-40.

20) Price JD, Sear JJ, Venn RR. Perioperative fluid volume optimization following proximal femoral fracture. Cochrane Database of Systematic Reviews. 2004(1).

21) Elbashier OE, Hamza AA. Postoperative Fluid Management in Emergency Abdominal Surgery in Omdurman Teaching Hospital. Gezira Journal of Health Sciences. 2019; 15:1.

22) Strunden MS, Heckel K, Goetz AE, Reuter DA. Perioperative fluid and volume management: physiological basis, tools and strategies. Annals of intensive care. 2011 Dec; 1:1-8.

23) Doherty M, Buggy DJ. Intraoperative fluids: how much is too much? British journal of anaesthesia. 2012 Jul 1;109(1):69-79.

24) Bagshaw SM, Chawla LS. Hydroxyethyl starch for fluid resuscitation in critically ill patients. Canadian Journal of Anesthesia/Journal canadien d'anesthésie. 2013 Jul; 60:709-13.

25) Myburgh JA, Mythen MG. Resuscitation fluids. New England Journal of Medicine. 2013 Sep 26;369(13):1243-51.

26) Carson JL, Brooks MM, Abbott JD, Chaitman B, Kelsey SF, Triulzi DJ, Srinivas V, Menegus MA, Marroquin OC, Rao SV, Noveck H. Liberal versus restrictive transfusion thresholds for patients with symptomatic coronary artery disease. American heart journal. 2013 Jun 1;165(6):964-71.

27) Villanueva C, Colomo A, Bosch A, Concepción M, Hernandez-Gea V, Aracil C, Graupera I, Poca M, Alvarez-Urturi C, Gordillo J, Guarner-Argente C. Transfusion strategies for acute upper gastrointestinal bleeding. New England Journal of Medicine. 2013 Jan 3;368(1):11-21.

28) Caironi P, Tognoni G, Masson S, Fumagalli R, Pesenti A, Romero M, Fanizza C, Caspani L, Faenza S, Grasselli G, Iapichino G. Albumin replacement in patients with severe sepsis or septic shock. New England Journal of Medicine. 2014 Apr 10;370(15):1412-21.

29) Shim HJ, Jang JY, Lee SH, Lee JG. The effect of positive balance on the outcomes of critically ill noncardiac postsurgical patients: a retrospective cohort study. Journal of Critical Care. 2014 Feb 1;29(1):43-8.

30) Ettinger KS, Yildirim Y, Van Ess JM, Rieck KL, Viozzi CF, Arce K. Impact of intraoperative fluid administration on length of postoperative hospital stay following orthognathic surgery. Journal of Oral and Maxillofacial Surgery. 2015 Jan 1;73(1):22-9.

31) Kayilioglu SI, Dinc T, Sozen I, Bostanoglu A, Cete M, Coskun F. Postoperative fluid management. World journal of critical care medicine. 2015 Aug 8;4(3):192.

32) Saraghi M. Intraoperative fluids and fluid management for ambulatory dental sedation and general anesthesia. Anesthesia Progress. 2015 Dec 1;62(4):168-77.

33) Hariri F. Revisiting the basis of perioperative fluid management in oral and maxillofacial surgery. Malaysian Journal of Oral and Maxillofacial Surgery. 2016 Jan 1;14(1):8-12.

34) Wise R, Faurie M, Malbrain ML, Hodgson E. Strategies for intravenous fluid resuscitation in trauma patients. World journal of surgery. 2017 May; 41:1170-83.

35) Shin CH, Long DR, McLean D, Grabitz SD, Ladha K, Timm FP, Thevathasan T, Pieretti A, Ferrone C, Hoeft A, Scheeren TW. Effects of intraoperative fluid management on postoperative outcomes: a hospital registry study. Annals of surgery. 2018 Jun 1;267(6):1084-92.

36) Makaryus R, Miller TE, Gan TJ. Current concepts of fluid management in enhanced recovery pathways. British journal of anaesthesia. 2018 Feb 1;120(2):376-83.

37) Kang D, Yoo KY. Fluid management in perioperative and critically ill patients. Acute and Critical Care. 2019 Nov;34(4):235.

38) Miller TE, Myles PS. Perioperative fluid therapy for major surgery. Anesthesiology. 2019 May 1;130(5):825-32.

39) Heming N, Moine P, Coscas R, Annane D. Perioperative fluid management for major elective surgery. Journal of British Surgery. 2020 Jan;107(2): e56-62.

40) Brandstrup B, Møller AM. The challenge of perioperative fluid management in elderly patients. Current Anesthesiology Reports. 2019 Dec; 9:406-13.
41) Wiedermann CJ. Phases of fluid management and the roles of human albumin solution in perioperative and critically ill patients. Current medical research and opinion. 2020 Dec 1;36(12):1961-73.
42) Malbrain ML, Langer T, Annane D, Gattinoni L, Elbers P, Hahn RG, De Laet I, Minini A, Wong A, Ince C, Muckart D. Intravenous fluid therapy in the perioperative and critical care setting: executive summary of the International Fluid Academy (IFA). Annals of intensive care. 2020 Dec; 10:1-9.
43) Kamel RK, Shaboob EA, Youssef GS. New concepts in Perioperative Fluid Management. Benha Journal of Applied Sciences. 2021 Aug 1;6(4):163-8.
44) Koskinen A, Aittokallio J, Gunn J, Lehto J, Relander A, Viikinkoski E, Vasankari T, Jalkanen J, Hollmén M, Kiviniemi TO. Risk of fluid accumulation after cardiac surgery. JTCVS open. 2023 Dec 1; 16:602-9.
45) Hahn R, Reimsbach D, Wickert C. Nonfinancial reporting and real sustainable change: relationship status—it's complicated. Organization & Environment. 2023 Mar;36(1):3-16.
46) Koek S, Lo J, Ledger R, Ballal M. Postoperative fluid therapy in enhanced recovery after surgery for pancreaticoduodenectomy. Annals of hepato-biliary-pancreatic surgery. 2024 Feb 29;28(1):80-91.
47) Hahn RG, Van Regenmortel N. Is the NICE Guideline for Maintenance Fluid Therapy in Adults in Hospital appropriate? Clinical Nutrition ESPEN. 2024 Jun 19.
48) Hahn R, Reimsbach D, Wickert C. Nonfinancial reporting and real sustainable change: relationship status—it's complicated. Organization & Environment. 2023 Mar;36(1):3-16.
49) Karunarathna I, Kusumarathna K, Jayathilaka P, Withanagama C. Optimizing Fluid Management in Critical Care: Principles and Strategies. Uva Clinical Lab. Retrieved from Optimizing Fluid Management in Critical Care: Principles and Strategies. 2024.

50) Pandey CK, Singh R. Fluid and electrolyte disorders. Indian J Anaesth. 2013;47(5):380

51) Leonard SD, Lee JF. Hyponatremia and Syndrome of Inappropriate Antidiuretic Hormone after Orthopedic Surgery. Proceedings of UCLA Healthcare; 2017. Vol 21

52) Braun MM, Barstow CH, Pyzocha NJ. Diagnosis and management of sodium disorders: hyponatremia and hypernatremia. Am Fam Physician. 2015;91(5):299-307.

53) Viera AJ, Wouk N. Potassium disorders: hypokalemia and hyperkalemia. Am Fam Physician. 2015;92(6):487-95.

54) Bhardwaj B, Desai AD, Patel BM, Parekh CD, Patel SM. Prevalence of hypomagnesemia in patients undergoing gynecological oncology surgery in tertiary care cancer institute of India. Int J Reprod Contracept Obstet Gynecol. 2017;6(10):4355-62

55) Deheinzelin D, Negri EM, Tucci MR, Salem MZ, da Cruz VM, Oliveira RM, et al. Hypomagnesemia in critically ill cancer patients: a prospective study of predictive factors. Braz J Med Biol Res. 2000;33(12):1443-8

56) Brainard BM, Campbell VL, Drobatz KJ, Perkowski SZ. The effects of surgery and anesthesia on blood magnesium and calcium concentrations in canine and feline patients. Vet Anaesth Analg. 2007;34(2):89-98

57) Walker MD. Fluid and electrolyte imbalances: interpretation and assessment. J Infus Nurs. 2016;39(6):382-6

58) Lowry SF. Fluid, Electrolyte, and Acid-Base Disorders in the Surgery Patient. In: Lowry SF, Ciocca RG, Rettie CS, Vodarsik M, eds. Learning Surgery. New York, NY: Springer; 2005. p. 62-81

59) RANDALL RE Jr, PAPPER S. Mechanism of postoperative limitation in sodium excretion: the role of extracellular fluid volume and of adrenal cortical activity. J Clin Invest. 1958;37(11):1628-1641

60) Gennari FJ. Disorders of potassium homeostasis. Hypokalemia and hyperkalemia. Crit Care Clin. 2002;18(2):273-88, vi.

61) Kamoun S, Alves A, Bretagnol F, Lefevre JH, Valleur P, Panis Y. Outcomes of laparoscopic colorectal surgery in obese and nonobese patients: a case-matched study of 180 patients. Am J Surg. 2009;198(3):450-5

62) Thomas EJ, Goldman L, Mangione CM, Marcantonio ER, Cook EF, Ludwig L, et al. Body mass index as a correlate of postoperative complications and resource utilization. Am J Med. 1997;102(3):277-83

63) American Society of Anesthesiologist Task Force (1999) Practice guidelines for preoperative fasting and the use of pharmacologic agents to reduce the risk of pulmonary aspiration: application to healthy patients undergoing elective procedures: a report by the American Society of Anesthesiologist Task Force on PreoperativeFasting. Anesthesiology 90:896-905

64) Reid F, Lobo DN, Williams RN, Rowlands BJ, Allison SP (2003) (Ab)normal saline and physiological Hartmann's solution: a randomized double-blind crossover study. Clin Sci (Lond) 104:17-24.

65) Morgan GE, Mikhail MS Jr), Murray MJ (2005) Clinical Anathesiology 4th edn. McGraw-Hill Professional Publishing, pp690-70

66) Pandya S (2002) Practical Guidelines on Fluid Therapy, 2 ed. Bhalani Book House, Mumbai (India) Pp 262-285 34.

67) Brandstrup B, Tønnesen H, Beier-Holgersen R, et al. Effects of intravenous fluid restriction on postoperative complications: comparison of two perioperative fluid regimens: a randomized assessor-blinded multicenter trial. Ann Surg. 2003;238(5):641–8

68) Kulemann B, Timme S, Seifert G, et al. Intraoperative crystalloid overload leads to substantial inflammatory infiltration of intestinal anastomoses—a histomorphological analysis. Surg (United States). 2013;154(3):596–603

69) Neal JM, Wilcox RT, Allen HW, Low DE. Near-total esophagectomy: the influence of standardized multimodal management and intraoperative fluid 64 Fluid and Electrolyte therapy in OMFS restriction. Reg Anesth Pain Med. 2003;28(4):328–34.

70) National Heart and Blood Institute Acute Respiratory Distress Syndrome (ARDS) Clinical Trials Network L. Comparison of two fluid-management strategies in acute lung injury. N Engl J Med. 2006;354:2564–75.

71) Marjanovic G, Villain C, Juettner E, et al. Impact of different crystalloid volume regimes on intestinal anastomotic stability. Ann Surg. 2009;249(2): 181–5. doi:10.1097/SLA.0b013e31818b73d

72) Henriksen MG, Hessov I, Dela F, Hansen HV, Haraldsted V, Rodt SA. Effects of preoperative oral carbohydrates and peptides on postoperative endocrine response, mobilization, nutrition and muscle function in abdominal surgery. Acta Anaesthesiol Scand. 2003;47(2): 191–9

73) Soop M, Nygren J, Myrenfors P, Thorell A, Ljungqvist O. Preoperative oral carbohydrate treatment attenuatesimmediate postoperative insulin resistance. Am J Physiol Endocrinol Metab. 2001;280(4):E576–83

74) Jacob M, Chappell D, Conzen P, Finsterer U, Rehm M. Blood volume is normal after pre-operative overnight fasting. Acta Anaesthesiol Scand. 2008; 52(4):522–9. doi:10.1111/j.1399-6576.2008.01587.x.

75) Holte K. Pathophysiology and clinical implications of peroperative fluid management in elective surgery. Dan Med Bull. 2010;57(7):B4156.

76) Reithner L. Insensible water loss from the respiratory tract in patients with fever. Acta Chir Scand. 1981;147(3):163–7.

77) de Aguilar-Nascimento JE, Diniz BN, do Carmo AV, Silveira EAO, Silva RM. Clinical benefits after the implementation of a protocol of restricted perioperative intravenous crystalloid fluids in major abdominal operations. World J Surg. 2009;33(5):925–30.

78) Hall, J. E. (2015). Guyton and hall textbook of medical physiology (13th ed.). W B Saunders.

79) Williams NS, Bullstrode CJK, O'Connell PR. Bailey & Love's Short Practice of Surgery, 25th edn. Ann R Coll Surg Engl. 2010 Mar;92(2):178

80) A manual on clinical surgery. Second edition. S. Das. 182 × 248 mm. Pp. 398. Illustrated. 1987. Calcutta: Dr S. Das

Kolibri 360 GmbH
Ferdinand-Jühlke-Straße 7
99095 Erfurt, Deutschland
produktsicherheit@kolibri360.de

Druck:
CPI Druckdienstleistungen GmbH
im Auftrag der
Kolibri 360 GmbH
Ferdinand-Jühlke-Str. 7
99095 Erfurt